UNDERSTANDING POSTMODERN FAMILY THERAPY

W0018714

This accessible textbook provides therapy students and practitioners with an understanding of postmodern theories, founders, and practical applications to family therapy. It introduces complex concepts in bite-sized pieces so readers can cultivate and master competent real-world applications of postmodern philosophy in therapy.

Relying predominantly on primary sources, Kelsey Railsback shows how postmodernist ideas influenced the development and implementation of postmodern family therapy models, focusing on collaborative-dialogic practice, narrative therapy, and solution focused brief therapy. It describes why certain therapeutic techniques developed and explains the context and history of their development. Each section begins with an introduction to the model before moving to the philosopher and ending with the founders' application of philosophical ideas to therapy techniques. These chapters summarize prominent ideas from esteemed professionals in their fields, covering the philosophical pioneers Wittgenstein, Foucault, and Gergen and the therapy pioneers Anderson, White, Epston, de Shazer, Berg, and more. Critically, this book demonstrates how postmodern theory can be applied in mental health practice. By the end of the book, students will be able to interweave the philosophers, founders, and applications of postmodern family therapy into a comprehensive picture. To better understand their epistemology and why they are more inclined toward certain practices over others, students can utilize the included self-quizzes to deepen their understanding.

Filled with etymological explanations, reflective questions, keywords, and summaries throughout, this book is designed for students and practitioners in systemic and relational therapy or related fields such as psychology, social work, and mental health counseling.

Kelsey Railsback, Ph.D., LMFT, is an AAMFT Approved Supervisor and a core faculty member at Touro University Worldwide. She provides classroom instruction and oversees clinical supervision of master's and doctoral students in Marriage and Family Therapy.

Understanding Postmodern Family Therapy

Interweaving Theory and Applying Models in Context

Kelsey Railsback

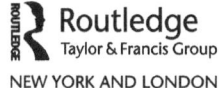

Routledge
Taylor & Francis Group

NEW YORK AND LONDON

Designed cover image: © Nathan Lewis

First published 2025
by Routledge
605 Third Avenue, New York, NY 10158

and by Routledge
4 Park Square, Milton Park, Abingdon, Oxon, OX14 4RN

Routledge is an imprint of the Taylor & Francis Group, an informa business

© 2025 Kelsey Railsback

ISBN: 9781032574363 (hbk)
ISBN: 9781032574349 (pbk)
ISBN: 9781003439349 (ebk)

DOI: 10.4324/9781003439349

Typeset in Sabon
by KnowledgeWorks Global Ltd.

Contents

Dedication

This book is dedicated to the memory of Dr. William C. Rambo, whose presence still lingers in the spaces between these words. A staunch advocate of the Mental Research Institute (MRI), I can almost hear his grumbles about postmodern practices echoing through these pages. And yet it was through his modernist guidance that I began to find myself as a postmodern therapist as he connected me to Harlene Anderson's collaborative-dialogic practice (C-DP). I can imagine him shaking his head at my words, which are essentially a love letter to C-DP, and yet I know he would have begrudgingly admired the effort nonetheless. I will continue to cherish our conversations about philosophy, ontology, theology, and activism. In remembrance of a cherished mentor, this book is a testament to his lasting impact.

Author introduction

Kelsey Railsback, Ph.D., is a core faculty member at Touro University Worldwide. She provides classroom instruction and oversees clinical supervision of master's and doctoral students in Marriage and Family Therapy. She is a licensed marriage and family therapist (LMFT), Qualified Supervisor (QS), American Association for Marriage and Family Therapy (AAMFT) Clinical Fellow, AAMFT Approved Supervisor, and international life coach. She also serves as the Director of Ethics on the Advisory Board of the Low-Cost Community Counseling Center, a non-profit mental health center in Sante Fe Springs, California, "where compassionate support meets affordability." Her professional interests include qualitative research and working with marginalized populations.

Dr. Railsback earned her master's and doctoral degrees in Family Therapy from Nova Southeastern University. She is deeply passionate about understanding the philosophy that influenced the founders' development and application of their family therapy models. Although fond of a few modernist family therapy models, she overwhelmingly prefers postmodern family therapy practices.

Dr. Railsback's unique bachelor's degree comes from St. John's College, where she double-majored in Philosophy and the History of Mathematics and Science and double-minored in Classical Studies and Comparative Literature. Dr. Railsback's unconventional learning environment prepared her to approach ideas in family therapy in unique and varied ways. For example, learning ancient Greek to translate and better understand Plato and Aristotle is not a common college requirement.

Preface

The idea for this book first occurred to me during my master's program. I noticed my peers and colleagues were less interested in the history or epistemology of the family therapy models and preferred to focus on the "how-to" of therapeutic application. Peers were far more interested in what questions they should ask, how to write notes, and how to work with insurance. These are undoubtedly critical procedural aspects; however, focusing on practical knowledge need not eliminate interest in theoretical knowledge.

In my doctoral program, I became an unofficial tutor, explaining to my peers why the epistemological foundations shaped the model and why a misunderstanding of the epistemology would lead to a misapplication of the model and its techniques. Such discussions were filled with laughter and teasing one another over what models we thought we "were." Our conversations would often lead to different understandings of the model and ourselves.

After graduation, I taught a master's course on postmodernism in family therapy. I realized that my prior experience as a "postmodern" "philosopher" could be incredibly valuable to students who grew up in a modernist world. My penchant for quotation marks around every other word took some getting used to, but my students came to appreciate the tentative and skeptical nature of postmodern thought. They came to mirror a view of labels as provisional and see them as tentatively useful, not universally absolute.

Later, I taught practicum supervision for interns in marriage and family therapy where I heard, "You should write a book about this" followed by, "Nobody knows this" too many times to count. I responded, saying this information was out there if only one knew where to look. Eventually, I realized I was repeating the same primary source reading recommendations and my interpretations of them ad infinitum. The idea of writing a book, synthesizing the information in one place, was born of passion, certainly, but catalyzed by a desire to save time.

As I was writing this text, I struggled with how many philosophers to include. One way to have done it would have been to focus on every philosopher who influenced a founder, but there would have been an intermingling of epistemologies that would have made the text convoluted and taken it away from its postmodern purpose.

A second way would have been to focus on the one philosopher that influenced a founder "the most," but that would have necessarily needed a lot of caveats since people are (more often than not) influenced by many voices. A third way would be to focus on the influential philosophers to which different postmodernist family therapy founders kept referring. I wrote this text each of those ways before metaphorically tearing up the pages and starting anew. This fourth way focuses on the postmodern philosopher—or philosopher associated with postmodernism, as it were—that the founders were enamored by and whose influence can be seen when their model's techniques are employed. Thus this book does not cover every philosophic and theoretical influence on a family therapy founder. Perhaps I will write that book in the future.

I imagine this is the sort of book that a student will start to read in the manner of my old peers: as a "how-to." However, I think this book can help students and interns discover "what model they 'are'" by discovering how they think, what they believe in, and what they value—in addition to learning how to carry out a model according to the founders themselves. It is not that every word in this book is significant. But every word, comma, and semi-colon was thoughtfully chosen to convey a particular meaning. For example, every sentence ending in a preposition, a metaphorical arrow to my heart, is a decision made with conscious attention and intention to make this book more accessible for students and interns striving to balance their studies, jobs, and families. The goal of this book is not to impress but to inform, or rather, to inspire.

I love philosophy, ethics, metaphysics, linguistics, etymology, mythology, theology, and social justice. And I feel the most "me" working from a postmodern stance. Postmodern family therapy has become another love of mine. If you read this book and hate all the postmodern ideas you read, that is okay. At least you will have become more aware of what you *do* believe in and *why*. A gracious student recently told me,

> While I don't share many of your inclinations and biases, I find them valuable, and I feel the freedom to fully develop my own. You always get me thinking about the material and inspire me to understand why I do what I do, as well as other approaches.
>
> *(Student G)*

Perfect.

Understanding Postmodern Family Therapy: Interweaving Theory and Applying Models in Context connects each model with its underlying epistemology. It is designed for master's and doctoral students and interns in family therapy or related fields such as psychology, social work, and mental health counseling. Seasoned therapists who want to deepen their understanding of postmodern practices will also find a valuable companion in this book. By introducing complex concepts in bite-sized pieces, readers can cultivate a deep understanding and build competence in a real-world application. Some academics have written off postmodernism entirely, and some think it is wildly outrageous in psychotherapy. To understand postmodern ideas, one must step outside the modernist comfort zone. Adopt a stance of curiosity rather than an argumentative, dismissive, or acrimonious internal dialogue. This book acknowledges the controversy of radical ideas that challenge dominant discourses and seeks to embrace discussions of differences that shift the human experience.

Notes to the reader

1. There is an author and family therapist, Tom Andersen (with an "e"), as well as another author and family therapist named Harlene Anderson (with an "o"). I say this to avoid confusion when they both have works in the same year. For example, "(Anderson, 2012)" and "(Andersen, 2012)" may both be present; neither is a typo.
2. There is something called "*withness* practice" (see Andersen, Anderson, or Hoffman) and something else called "outsider *witness* practice" (see White); neither is a typo.
3. There is a concept called "both/and," which is contrasted to "either/or," and these family therapy terms are used in ways that may otherwise seem odd to the everyday reader.
4. Unusual capitalization and pluralization are present and intentional. At times, there will be words used in ways that may surprise you such as "knowledges" and "Truth."
5. The Preface is in the front matter, while the Introduction is a section of **Part I**.
6. Narrative therapist marcela polanco prefers a lowercase spelling, so the APA 7 citation would be, for instance: Monk, G., Winslade, J., Sinclair, S., & **polanco, m.** (2020). *Intercultural counseling: Bridging the us and them divide* (1st ed.). Cognella.
7. In the solution focused brief therapy section, De Jong will be capitalized; meanwhile, de Shazer will have a lowercase "d."
8. *Solution focused brief therapy* used to be "solution-focused brief therapy," but the model lost its hyphen over time.

Acknowledgments

I am sincerely thankful for the dedicated faculty, staff, and fellow students who have contributed to my education and personal development during my master's and doctoral careers at Nova Southeastern University, notably Francesca Angiuli, Christine Beliard, Charmaine Borda, Arlene Brett Gordon, James Hibel, Martha Marquez, and Anne Rambo.

To my esteemed mentors—Limor Ast, Ron Chenail, Kara Erolin, Douglas Flemons, Shelley Green, and Michael D. Reiter—your guidance, wisdom, and expertise have been invaluable to me. Thank you for sharing your knowledge, insights, and passion for the field. I am indebted to each of you for your mentorship and friendship.

Limor, your candid way of being and passionate introduction to narrative therapy fueled me to strive to "be like you when I grow up." Your trust in my lived experience allowed me to trust myself as a therapist. Your way of being is inimitable, and your reading recommendations are treasured. As I see it, "growing up" will be about 50 years from now. It will be worth the wait.

Ron, thank you for seeing me as my future self and providing me with the resources to get there. Your mentorship is the closest thing I have experienced to a utopian meritocracy. I loved becoming a copyeditor, production editor, conference moderator, guest speaker, and qualitative researcher under your tutelage. I could talk to you for days and never notice it was longer than 15 minutes. And I got to attend Ken Gergen's lecture because of you, which was a nice TQR bonus.

Kara, I learned to put words to feelings under your guidance as I found my footing in social justice issues. Your mentorship has allowed me to work ethically with marginalized populations and believe in myself, standing by my values. You also gave me new insights into trauma work and how I can be more present with clients.

Douglas, you have been a model for how playfulness and humor can be ethically incorporated into sessions. The seriousness with which you approach the craft of therapy and your creativity are inspiring. You have been influential in helping me see the world more relationally despite the cultural and linguistic pulls of North American English.

Shelley, your mentorship allowed me to get in touch with myself. You endlessly demonstrate warmth, acceptance, and the ability to "meet people where they are at." I would not have had my life-changing experience working with sex offenders had you not made such a dramatic impact on my life (I know, not the most Batesonian language) and understanding of human sexuality and social justice.

Michael, it takes some supervisory know-how to turn my contribution of Rage Against the Machine lyrics into something therapeutically relevant. I cherish that memory. Thank you for joining my sarcasm and making room for my ethics, morality, agnosticism, and endless figurative taps on the shoulder. I will very likely never do what you tell me, but I will very likely always value your opinion.

Teachers hardly get the recognition they deserve, and I was able to write this book because of a series of English and writing teachers who believed in me, starting in elementary school. I want to express immense gratitude for the educational support and unconditional positive regard from Mrs. Schultz, Mrs. Mullaney, Mrs. Newman, Mrs. Birr, and Mr. Jaswinski. In second grade, Mrs. Schultz taught me to enjoy reading. In fifth grade, Mrs. Mullaney taught me to avoid ending sentences in prepositions, which unfortunately happens in this book. Sorry, Mrs. Mullaney. In sixth grade, Mrs. Newman taught me the wonder of semicolons, regardless of Kurt Vonnegut's scorn. In high school, Mrs. Birr taught me to allow literature to awaken parts of myself. I am grateful for the encouragement I received from these women. I am also indebted to my Latin instructor, Mr. Jaswinski, for instilling a somewhat-problematic-but-often-affirming veneration for languages, etymology, and grammar.

I am again grateful for Drs. Ron Chenail and Douglas Flemons for teaching me to break all the grammatical rules I thought I knew. I have rewritten my "to-write" list with your influence. It stands as follows: Don't try to sound academic, replace professional language with local language, and feel free to start sentences with conjunctions as long as you do not place a comma immediately after them. I have tried my best to incorporate your refinements. Ron, I apologize for starting sentences with "therefore." I know you would prefer the sentence to be structured like this; however, I was not always able to do so. Douglas, thank you for reinforcing that semicolons *are* magical and allow the reader to draw their own conclusions rather than have the author spell out the relation between two sentences. You both have renewed my appreciation for the difference between metaphors and similes. And I can see how semicolons as less directive than conjunctions. I understand this is usually overlooked; it matters greatly to me.

I am profoundly grateful to my life partner, travel companion, and favorite artist. Nathan, you have been endearingly "accidentally Narrative," soliciting my *sparkling moments* and *thickening the story* of my *preferred narrative*. I also appreciate that you, even as "a man of science," make space for me and my continuous postmodern critiques of the "Scientification of knowledge(s)." Over the years, your openness and support have transformed my life into a total experience instead of a *totalizing experience*.

I would also like to express my appreciation for my "conversational partners": Adrian, Akiva, Alessandro, Allana, Antonette, Ariadna, Ariela, Arthrine, Aubrey, Bailee, Benjamin, Boris, Breanne, Brenda, Brittany, Brooke, Cailin, Carol, Carrie, Cecilia, Chris, Christina, Daniel, Dane, Dorcas, Erin, Farhad, Giancarlo, Graham, Ivan, Jacqueline, Jessica, Jessie, Johnathan, Jonathan, Julie, Kimberley, Laura, Lisa, Liz, Luke, Marcelle, Marissa, Mario, Martin, Michaela, Mike, Nadia, Paula, Peter,

Pierre, Pooja, Quinnett, Rafis, Raquel, Ryan, Sabrina, Sara, Sarah, Shar, Shauneequa, Simona, Solomon, Stacii, Stefano, Stevie, Sylvia, Teline, Thomas, Warren, and Zara. Our transformative dialogues have enriched my understanding and fueled my creativity. My life is better because of our conversations.

A special appreciation goes to my "book doula" Judith Russell and "book midwife" Beth Hannan-Abesamis. Judith, your nurturing support and insightful feedback from idea development to the final manuscript have been invaluable. Beth, your dedication to comments and edits, despite your busy schedule, has elevated the quality of this book immensely. A special thanks also goes out to my copyeditor, Paula, for making this project successful in meeting its deadline.

To my family—Debbie, Patrick, Scott, Diana, Ed, and Georgette—your patient ears and unwavering support have been a source of strength. Thank you for tolerating my endless musings on the "-logys" and the "-isms" that made their way into this book (e.g., epistemology, ontology, constructivism, and social constructionism). Your love and encouragement have been a guiding light on this journey.

Lastly, my time at St. John's College has been invaluable, so I would like to thank my tutors and fellow Johnnies for providing a cherished academic environment. Go platypuses/axolotls! This inevitably leads me back to thanking my family for supporting my dream to attend such a unique program. That once-in-a-lifetime educational experience has certainly made me a better therapist and, I like to think, a better person.

PART I

Introduction

GETTING STARTED

A quick internet search reveals that psychology is the study of the mind and behavior. However, let us examine the origin of "psychology." The etymology of psychology comes from the ancient Greek roots PSUKHE (ψυχή, pronounced "soo-kay") + LOGOS (λόγος, pronounced "low-gowz"). *Psukhe* means "soul," and *logos* has many meanings but is often translated as "to know" or "the study of." Thus *psychology* started as a philosophical inquiry concerned with the study of the soul.

Perhaps you are more familiar with the Latinized version of *"psukhe,"* which is *"psyche"* (pronounced "sigh-kee"). Those familiar with the Roman myth will recall that Cupid falls in love with and marries Psyche, creating a union between love and soul. I share this etymological and mythological information to shed light on how much Western mental health practices have shifted over time away from "the study of the soul."

To find *psukhe*, we can look to the great Greek orator Homer and to the Christian Bible. Homer's work in *The Iliad* and *The Odyssey* introduced *psukhe* as soul, spirit, or life-breath and described a man dying as the *psukhe* leaving his body (Cairns, 2015, para. 11). Common Biblical translations of *psukhe* include soul, life, live, heart, heartily, person, soul-life, being, everyone, living creatures, and living thing (Chang, 2017, p. 265). The New Revised Standard Version of the Bible translates *psukhe* as "soul" 56 times and "mind" one time (Chang). "Mind" is not necessarily a wrong translation of *psukhe* but a fringe translation of the ancient Greek word.

If we can agree, as Steve de Shazer (1991) did, that the best translation of *psukhe* is soul and *psychology* = SOUL + STUDY OF, how did we come to believe psychology is the study of the mind? To make a philosopher's pun, we put "De Cartes before the horse." René Descartes (pronounced "Ruh-nay Day-Kaart") propagated a new way of thinking during the Age of Reason, leaving behind the ancient Greek word "psukhe" in favor of its Latin derivative, "psyche."

I believe languages shape how we think. Although Descartes was a French philosopher, he often thought and wrote in Latin to make his work more academically

DOI: 10.4324/9781003439349-1

acceptable and accessible. You are likely familiar with Descartes' quote: "Cogito, ergo sum," frequently translated into English as "I think, therefore I am."

You know as well as I do that words take on a part of the culture in which they are used. When you are translating a language into other languages, you are not just changing the word but the context, meaning, and philosophy behind it. And, sometimes, meaning gets "lost in translation." Descartes' use of the Latin *psyche* became intertwined with his modernist way of thinking called empiricism (discussed elsewhere in the Introduction). Descartes' philosophy introduced a division between soul and body, named *Cartesian dualism* after him. This division of mind and body has permeated psychology since then. The meaning of psychology in this empiricist context is hyper-rationalism. In other words, philosophizing about the soul shifted to "scientific" observation and attempts at measuring the brain or mind, as we see today. This change is illustrated well by the juxtaposition of Socrates' quote: "The unexamined life is not worth living," with Descartes' quote: "I think, therefore I am." Psychology moved from the Platonic (i.e., referring to Plato)-ancient Greek understanding of "soul" to the Cartesian-Latin understanding of "mind." Western society shifted from philosophy toward one of philosophy's original subsets, science, moving from a focus on description to a focus on "rational" explanation. Whereas the first emphasized contemplation, the second emphasized investigation. One might say the former focused on a quest for living well, and the latter focused on a quest for information.

Cartesian dualism separates us into parts that we analyze. But ask yourself, why are we married to the idea that we are lumps of organs (i.e., body) + a computer (i.e., a mind)? Where did we learn this idea from? And does more analysis equal happier living? Think of how often we are taught that "mental health" addresses mental "disease" and mirrors physical health and physical disease. This book, being a postmodern family therapy book, holds a critique of Cartesian dualism and the medicalization of the soul. This does not imply a complete disregard for scientific inquiry. Rather, it encourages an acknowledgment that Western society, over the centuries, has leaned into a reification of science which has marginalized alternative ways of living (e.g., those found in indigenous cultures). Postmodernism critiques the resulting reductive view and sees it as an eclipse of the human experience. Therefore, this book, and postmodernism in general, is not for everyone. Much of the information may contradict knowledge that students have been taught in classes and passed on exams. I hope the differentness of postmodern practices does not dissuade you from taking it seriously, as there are many benefits to a postmodern stance in therapy.

THEORY AND PRACTICE: THE AIM AND STRUCTURE OF THIS BOOK

One topic that may be difficult for students, interns, or even practicing psychotherapists to grasp is the relationship between philosophy and therapy. Frequently, learners memorize the names of relevant philosophers to pass a class, but they rarely develop a depth of understanding regarding each philosopher's ideas. After reading this book, you will be able to make connections to see how philosophy and theoretical orientations influence therapy and a therapist's practice.

This book aims to help mental health practitioners, interns, and students better see how philosophy shapes therapy in much the same way different colors of thread come together to form a rich tapestry, each color contributing to the overall design. We dive into philosophical theories, focusing on the philosophers whose ideas resonated with the founders of three major postmodern family therapy models: collaborative-dialogic practice (C-DP), narrative therapy, and solution focused brief therapy (SFBT).

These models are presented from most to least postmodern, opening with C-DP and closing with SFBT. As time progressed, postmodern ideas gained more traction in family therapy. Since the structure of this book is dictated by family therapy's historical and socio-cultural shifts, the models are thus also arranged in reverse chronological order.

Consequently, you will find the SFBT section contains less information than the C-DP section because SFBT has less of a foundation in postmodernism. As I explain in the SFBT section of this book, Insoo Kim Berg and Steve de Shazer's model originated from the hypnotherapist Milton Erickson and from modernist practices at the Mental Research Institute (MRI) in Palo Alto. Because of this, SFBT could be referred to as a "bridge model," starting in modernism but incorporating elements of postmodernism as time progressed.

Although SFBT is frequently identified as a social constructionist model (Bannink, 2007), this is a complicated issue since Berg and de Shazer were practicing before these co-founders were aware of Ken Gergen's ideas on social constructionism and even before de Shazer came across Ludwig Wittgenstein, whose ideas influenced the development of postmodernism but certainly preceded the development of social constructionism. However, the bright side of having a modernist foundation is that it is an easier foundation for an evidence-based model. SFBT is often said to be the only postmodern, systemic family therapy model that is evidence-based—although narrative therapy and C-DP have growing research to support efficacy and, as Harlene Anderson pointedly said, "Like collaborative and narrative therapies, the effectiveness of solution focused therapy is mostly found in anecdotal and specific case reports" (2016, p. 198).

It should become clear by the end of this book, if not the end of this paragraph, that it is easier to have your model recognized as evidence-based if it has a modernist base. Even though it is no secret that the co-founders of SFBT were not fond of SFBT being manualized as a recipe of questions, when a model is manualized, questions and techniques can be isolated and repeated by many practitioners. Thus SFBT has been identified as evidence-based, and "its techniques/questions are empirically supported change agents" (Chenail et al., 2020, p. 421). In a society where modernism dominates, the more postmodern a model is, the less likely it is to be evidence-based (according to traditional definitions and understandings). The less formulaic a model is, the harder it is to replicate. But this says more about our means of measurement than it does about a model's efficacy. Do not conflate "evidence-based" with "effective." Research's connection to modernism and postmodernism will become clearer as you learn more throughout this book.

Before you begin your journey to understanding postmodern family therapy, consider your answers to the questions in the Pre-Test below. Your answers may help you determine your personal philosophy of therapeutic practice, enabling you to better understand why certain models resonate with you. This will refine your understanding of yourself and the models you are drawn to. At a minimum, your answers will inform whether modernist or postmodernist models are a better fit for you. You may also want to return to these questions at the end of this book to see if your answers have changed. I believe knowing your answers to these questions is essential to ethical practice.

PRE-TEST

1. What is the role of a therapist?
2. What is the goal of a therapist?
3. How do you think change happens in therapy?
4. Should a therapist give advice?
5. How does a therapist find out what the problem is?
6. Should a therapist give homework?
7. What should a therapist do if a client fails to do their homework?
8. Should therapists self-disclose information about themselves?
9. What should a therapist's treatment plan look like?
10. At what point is a client non-compliant?
11. How close should a therapist be to their clients? How close is too close?
12. What is the function of language in therapy?
13. Should a therapist use "we" language?
14. When should a therapist terminate sessions?
15. How does a therapist know whether therapy is successful?

KEY INFORMATION: EXPLANATION OF TERMS

Family therapists and other mental health professionals are almost exclusively taught therapy models that fall under one of two categories: (1) **modern** or (2) **postmodern**, which I will soon explain. Students in Western education systems, particularly in psychotherapy programs, are predominantly taught to see the world from a modernist lens. This usually means they practice modernist models more frequently, leading to confusion and misapplication when postmodern models are introduced. "Operationalized" refers to creating a "how-to" that, quite frankly, misses the point, taking models out of their philosophical context. Often, when postmodern therapy models are introduced to modernist-practiced thinkers, they mistakenly seek to operationalize the models through "techniques" rather than take time to gather the context needed to understand the complete picture.

To correct this common misunderstanding, postmodern family therapy founders such as Harlene Anderson, Michael White, and Steve de Shazer explained the importance of the philosophers who influenced their therapeutic work: Ken Gergen, Michel Foucault, and Ludwig Wittgenstein, respectively (see Anderson, 1997; de Shazer et al., 2021; White & Epston, 1990). However, many students do not understand the significance of this and skim over the history, philosophy, and necessary background information. Many students frantically try to figure out what questions to ask clients rather than explore why or how they should be asking them.

As a philosophy major with an MFT license and PhD in Family Therapy, I see the value of keeping the philosophy close to the models. This book encourages the deep comprehension needed for postmodern practice in coursework and clinics. Part I introduces key terms.

What is modernism?

Modernism and postmodernism refer to two separate philosophical movements which differ significantly in their beliefs, practices, and underlying principles. *Modernism* is a complex term for a historical, cultural, intellectual, and artistic movement of the early 20th century, so it is hard to pin down a specific set of characteristics; however, in our context, you can think of modernism as the "traditional" approaches in psychology, philosophy, and research. Modernist psychological and research practices suggest there is a "correct" and "incorrect" way to understand a concept, do an activity, or draw a conclusion. Within a modernist lens of psychology, there is a right diagnosis and a wrong one; within family therapy, there is a right approach and a wrong one; and within research, there is a right methodology and a wrong one. In postmodernism, it is important to explore each individual's relationship to their diagnosis; there are many "right" approaches, some more helpful than others; there are many different kinds of research for different purposes. Modernism is the foil for postmodernism.

Modernism often aligns with a reinterpretation of tradition. Picasso, for example, was a modernist artist. Meanwhile, postmodernism is characterized by skepticism toward tradition or norms. Andy Warhol is an example of a well-known postmodern artist. Each philosophical stance has its own unique interdisciplinary implications.

> The modernist tradition refers to that movement of thought which originates with Descartes and which has perpetuated itself up to and into the twentieth century and seeks to realize philosophy's traditional goal of achieving a basic, fundamental knowledge of what is ... by turning inward, into the knowing subject himself ... where it seeks to discover grounds which will allow for certainty in our "knowledge" of "the external world."
>
> *(Madison, 1988, p. x, as cited in Anderson, 1997, p. 30)*

Modernism is an umbrella term that applies inside and outside the therapy room. It is "an approach to the understanding of events in the world that proposes it is possible *to directly know the world*—that it is possible for observers of certain phenomena to gain an *objective knowledge* of reality, of 'brute facts'" (White, 2011, pp. 149–150, as cited in Ilic, 2017, pp. 78–79, italics added for emphasis). Simply put, modernism assumes there is one Truth. (N.B.: In philosophy, capital letters are sometimes used to signify that the reader should interpret them differently than everyday usage; it tends to indicate the word is being used as an ultimate, absolute entity).

A modernist might conceptualize an individual as a metaphorical spelunker exploring caves and discovering more about the world "as it is." With postmodernism, an individual is not exploring but creating or co-creating, so there is no world "as it is" that can be accessed. Another way to say this is that in modernism, there is an assumed

"God's eye view" perspective that if we could only zoom out far enough, we would be able to see everything. "Everything," in this case, means the one true world or universe—one Truth. From a modernist lens, the more we know, the closer we get to Truth.

A modernist therapeutic approach reminds me of the Egyptian tale where the god Anubis would weigh an individual's heart after death to see if it was lighter than a feather. If the scale showed the person's heart was lighter than the Feather of Truth, they had done enough good to deserve to continue to the afterlife with the god Osiris. If not, their heart would be fed to a feared monster-goddess (Mark, 2018). I believe modernist psychotherapy models can tempt mental health practitioners into becoming arbiters of Truth and Justice. It can feel comforting to think you know what is truly happening in an individual, couple, or family. But what if there is no single Truth?

The consequences of this on psychotherapy are that a modernist mental health practitioner will often focus on figuring out what is *really* going on and employing the *right* intervention. This therapeutic process is a search for Truth in the form of a particular understanding of events and a localized problem followed by a fix-it procedure that is based on that perceived Truth (de Shazer et al., 2021). This modernist philosophy perpetuates the myths (according to my worldview) that a mental health practitioner is neutral, objective, unbiased, or an independent observer, often supposing themselves to be outside the family system. A family therapist coming from a modernist lens can be seduced into becoming a detective, lecturer, or judge of clients' experiences. The author is fully aware of her bias here—any lens that you have colors how you see the world.

What is postmodernism?

Postmodernism is an umbrella term for a movement predicated on a belief in multiple truths and can be understood as a reaction to and rejection of modernist ideas. The postmodern movement challenges traditional understandings established in modernist systems and societies.

> Postmodernism amplified skepticism. Postmodern adherents were a brilliant group of linguists and literary critics who were influenced by Ludwig Wittgenstein, Jacques Derrida, Michel Foucault, and Jean-Francois Lyotard. Put together, the effect of these writers' work was to undermine the Truth claims of philosophy, the objective standards of science, and the assumptions of social and psychological research.
>
> *(Hoffman, 2001, p. 17)*

Crucially, postmodernism challenges the idea of a singular reality. Controversially, a postmodern stance embraces a belief in multiple realities.

Postmodern practices rebel against the notion that there are absolute "correct" and "incorrect" approaches to, for example, creating art, raising a family, or engaging in a conversation. Postmodern family therapists are particularly interested in understanding the influence of context and culture. Postmodern practices make room for a multitude of voices, recognizing that individuals' experiences are influenced by various contextual factors such that we never reach a place where we are "neutral" or "without bias."

> In its simplest form, postmodernism refers to an ideological critique that departs radically from modernist traditions—in its questioning of the mono-voice modernist discourse as the overarching foundation of literary, political, and social thinking. Although there is no one postmodernism, in general it challenges the modernist notions of knowledge as objective and fixed, the knower and knowledge as independent of each other, language as representing truth and reality, and human nature as universal.
>
> *(Anderson & Burney, 1996)*

Understanding postmodernism requires a shift in one's thinking, or better yet, a change in the process of how one has usually been taught to think within the Western world. Postmodernism is a philosophical undertaking of skepticism toward modernist assumptions and the idea that there is only one Truth.

In a therapeutic setting, a postmodern family therapist's language evolves from focusing on what is *right* to focusing on what is *helpful*. To clarify, this does not mean that postmodernists are immoral and not concerned with right and wrong. Rather, a postmodern family therapist avoids thinking about an *absolute* right or wrong.

There is a different sort of curiosity that arises out of a postmodern therapeutic stance. Practicing family therapy from a postmodern stance can switch the spotlight from the therapist to the clients, exploring the clients' truths. I find postmodernism to be a humble philosophy wherein therapists are more concerned with what the *client* believes—and why. A postmodern family therapist would attune to what meaning a client makes from an experience more so than uncover what "actually" happened.

Postmodern family therapy certainly resonates with some more than others. It would be self-contradictory to claim that postmodern philosophy is the superior philosophy; it inarguably opens up possibilities for different ways of thinking. Just because I prefer a certain flavor of ice cream does not mean that flavor is the best and that everyone should agree it is the objectively best flavor. I suggest my readers avoid a combative questioning of whether postmodernism is *right*, which would miss the point. I emphatically borrow from Harlene Anderson and Diane Gehart (2023) when they opened their book with a thought-provoking proposition, "We invite you to consider the following: What does *any* orientation permit you to do and not do?" (p. 16, italics added for emphasis).

TABLE 0.1 Modern vs. postmodern views

Modernists	Postmodernists
• We can find, predict, and explain the world around us.	• We doubt we can find, predict, or explain "the world as it is."
• We can get closer to understanding reality.	• We believe in multiple realties.

What is social constructionism?

Social constructionism is a specific type of postmodern philosophy. "At the base of this social constructionist inquiry into meaning lies a simple and straightforward proposal: our understandings of the world—what we claim to be real, rational, and good—emerge from the social process in which we participate" (Gergen, 2023, p. 17). Bear with me as I break down these complex philosophies into bite-sized pieces.

Social constructionism and *radical constructivism* are types of postmodernism. Radical constructivism and social constructionism are distinct and should not be confused; each is a particular philosophy with its own beliefs. I continue this discussion in a later section as well. For now, I want to emphasize that the postmodern family therapy models I discuss in this book are each deemed a social constructionist model.

Not only would a social constructionist believe in multiple truths, which is the necessary assumption for postmodernism, but they would also believe that these multitudinous truths are constructed with others through language. Further, social constructionists believe this process takes place within a particular society, within a particular culture, and within a particular time. Family therapist Harlene Anderson summarized some critical social constructionist views below:

- language as formative rather than representative;
- knowledge as a communal achievement rather than an individual one;
- the observer as a participant in creating what is experienced or observed rather than an objective description; and
- self as a dynamic, relational social construct rather than a static individual, contained entity

(Anderson, 2023, p. 18)

For example, unlike modernist family therapist Salvador Minuchin, a social constructionist family therapist would not focus on addressing hierarchy or boundary issues. Unlike modernist family therapist Murray Bowen, the social constructionist family therapist would not be interested in triangulation or self-differentiation. Unlike modernist family therapist Jay Haley, the social constructionist family therapist would not attend to communication patterns or directives. In contrast to these modernist family therapy approaches, social constructionist family therapists would be interested in each family member's truths, realities, and worldviews.

FOUNDERS AND THEORIES OF POSTMODERN FAMILY THERAPY

The family therapy founders I discuss in this book are Harlene Anderson, Michael White, Insoo Kim Berg, and Steve de Shazer. Respectively, they contributed to collaborative-dialogic practice (formerly collaborative therapy), narrative therapy, and SFBT. Although more postmodern family therapy models certainly exist, I focus on the prominent postmodern models I see repeatedly in the classroom, in agencies, and on the licensure exam.

Why is philosophy important?

I have often been dumbstruck regarding how frequently the philosophical ideas underlying the models of C-DP, narrative therapy, and SFBT are dismissed and discarded; meanwhile, family therapists continually emphasize the importance of *context* in their therapeutic work. The philosophical underpinning *is* context. I wish to do more than highlight this point. I want to expand family therapists' understandings beyond what to do operationally to include why we do what we do, connecting practice with the philosophical underpinnings. I also believe that understanding why we use a technique changes how we do it.

In writing this book, I aim to refine readers' understanding of postmodern family therapy models. I hope to correct common misunderstandings of these models and their applications and techniques. I hope my readers will walk away with an appreciation of the philosophy that influenced the practices they use with their clients. And, yes, I fully see and embrace the irony of telling my readers how to implement postmodern models "the right way" since there is no absolute "right" in postmodernism.

I wrote most of this book using primary sources, meaning I cite the philosophers and postmodern family therapy founders themselves rather than what others have said they said. I like to avoid playing the "telephone" game in this way. However, I hope my readers will access the primary texts themselves and come to their own conclusions. I resonate with Wittgenstein's quote: "I should not like my writing to spare other people the trouble of thinking. But, if possible, to stimulate someone to thoughts of their own" (Wittgenstein, 1953/2009, p. 4).

ADDITIONAL QUESTIONS TO THINK ABOUT

1. Have you ever questioned how we perceive and understand the world around us?
2. What are your thoughts about how it might differ from one person to another?
3. Are you curious about the impact of our beliefs on our understandings of knowledge and reality?
4. How do you think our individual experiences shape our unique perspectives on the world?
5. Do you wonder about the role of culture, language, and norms in shaping our understanding?

EXPLORING EPISTEMOLOGICAL PARADIGMS

Welcome to the fascinating world of postmodern family therapy! Postmodernism has existed since the mid-20th century and gained a lot of pop culture attention in the 1960s. For example, a postmodern artist, Andy Warhol, took something simple, something taken for granted—a soup can—and started putting a unique spin on it with a new, rebellious artistic perspective. Postmodernists can be thought of as having a rebellious and creative spirit.

Postmodern family therapy practice took longer to gain a foothold in the mental health community because it was harder to measure success by the modernists' standards. For example, cognitive-behavioral therapy (CBT) is easy to measure by Step 1, Step 2, and Step 3. The founder of narrative therapy, Michael White, made a splash in the 1980s. Like Andy Warhol, Michael White just did it and people liked it. Warhol got a lot of criticism for making the soup can look different, and people were similarly criticizing Michael White because it was harder to measure client outcomes in narrative therapy (from a modernist lens). That is, until they saw how effective it was—even though it did not conform to the standards set by modernism. Today, these leaders of postmodernism in their respective fields, Warhol and White, are esteemed and admired.

MODERNISM AND POSTMODERNISM: SUMMARY

Modernism and postmodernism refer to two separate philosophical movements which differ significantly in their beliefs, practices, and underlying principles. Modernism often aligns with a reinterpretation of tradition. Picasso, for example, was a modernist artist. Meanwhile, postmodernism is characterized by skepticism toward tradition or norms. Andy Warhol is a renowned postmodern artist. Each philosophical stance has its own unique interdisciplinary implications.

> As a postmodernist, Warhol's entire artistic practice and persona stood, quite intentionally, in opposition to modernist ideas. He was the very antithesis of a Van Gogh, a Picasso, a Pollock. Where they (it was held) re-made the world visually and emotionally in the smithies of their tortured souls (to paraphrase James Joyce), Warhol blithely swiped subject matter from mass media. He presented himself as a kind of empty mirror for the images that were already all around us in advertising or entertainment or packaging. And his persona was famously cool and withdrawn, or even blank: just the opposite of the outsized, impassioned personalities of Picasso or Pollock.
>
> *(Sartwell, 2013, para. 4)*

BREAKING DOWN CONSTRUCTIVISM, RADICAL CONSTRUCTIVISM, AND SOCIAL CONSTRUCTIONISM

This section explores epistemological paradigms, focusing on *constructivism*, *radical constructivism*, and *social constructionism*. Each can be considered a lens through which to view the world. Each lens alters our considerations of the nature of knowledge and reality, as well as the role of subjective experience. Subsequently, this section addresses *positivism*, *empiricism*, and *post-positivism*, outlining their positions and relevance to modernist and postmodernist philosophies. This highlights their distinct views on objective truth, empirical evidence, and the subjectivity of research. I also acknowledge the "science wars" and the tension between modernist and postmodernist theories.

This information will be an informative and thought-provoking foundation for the models and philosophies discussed in this book. I encourage readers to reflect on their beliefs about knowledge, reality, and research. This will set the stage for a deeper understanding of the complexities within postmodern family therapy.

Most students often miss the definition of *epistemology* and its connection to how they see the world. Constructivism, radical constructivism, and social constructionism are all philosophies that deal with epistemology, which comes from the ancient Greek

EPISTEME (knowledge) + LOGOS (~to know). Roughly speaking, one's epistemology is what and how one knows what they think they know. An individual's epistemology is their personal philosophy of understanding the nature of knowledge. Consider the following epistemological questions:

1. What is knowledge?
2. How is knowledge acquired or produced?
3. What are the limits of knowledge?

Epistemology is closely related to *ontology*, which refers to what and how we know about existence. Ontology comes from the ancient Greek roots ONTOS (being) + LOGOS (~to know). Simplifying these concepts, epistemology deals with questions about knowledge, while ontology deals with questions about reality. Some ontological questions are:

1. What is the nature of reality?
2. Does God (or a universal being) exist?
3. Are there alternative realities?

Some examples of questions that are both epistemological and ontological are:

1. What is the relationship between knowledge and reality?
2. Do our beliefs about reality accurately represent it?
3. How does our knowledge change our understanding of the world?

Epistemology and ontology are key components in metaphysics and are the philosophical pillars of constructivism, radical constructivism, and social constructionism. As the etymology suggests, both construct*ivism* and social construct*ionism* are philosophies that view knowledge as a *construction*.

Aristotle introduced *metaphysics*, a branch of philosophy that comes from the ancient Greek roots META (beyond) + PHYSIKA (physics); therefore, it deals with things beyond the physical world. Metaphysics encompasses epistemology and ontology and deals with more abstract thinking. It may seem counterintuitive to challenge our classical understanding of knowledge and reality; however, this is not all speculative or reducible to "armchair philosophy." For example, metaphysics has enormous implications in quantum physics. Although quantum physics has empirical foundations, metaphysical discussions arise in interpreting the phenomena studied. Thus, from NASA astrophysicists to us common folk, we encounter physics and metaphysics in our daily lives.

Some examples of questions that are metaphysical are:

1. What is the relationship between mind and matter?
2. Is there a purpose or meaning to existence?
3. What is the fate of the universe?
4. Does life exist beyond Earth?
5. Do we live in a simulation?

Constructivism, radical constructivism, and social constructionism all touch upon metaphysical questions. This is complicated, but we will work through it together.

Constructivism is a lens that acknowledges reality exists "out there" but focuses on how an individual interprets that reality. A constructivist believes one can only know and interpret the world through one's own mental schemas based on previous experiences. Philosopher Ken Gergen said, "Constructivism places the origin of knowledge in the head of the individual" (2023, p. 40). Constructivist theory is often attributed to Piaget and Kelly (Anderson, 1997; Gergen, 2023), although Gergen (2023) pointed out that Plato, Descartes, and Kant had long before planted the seeds for constructivism to flourish.

Family therapist Harlene Anderson attributed constructivism's intense offspring—radical constructivism—to von Foerster, von Glasersfeld, Watzlawick, and Maturana (Anderson, 1997, p. 43). While constructivism acknowledges an external reality, albeit one filtered through subjective interpretations, *radical constructivism* is a more extreme lens that maintains question marks around any external reality "out there." They see knowledge as a product of the individual's mental processes and experiences. Although they do not outright deny an independent reality, radical constructivists are more *skeptical* about our ability to access or know it. Radical constructivism suggests that nothing can be understood as a thing in itself without our mind as a generative filter, so we cannot know the outside world in any objective or absolute sense. Everything we think we know is a construct. Radical constructivists do not necessarily negate the possibility of an external reality but question whether humans can ever have direct access to it.

In summary, to a constructivist, there is an external reality that exists independently but is filtered through our subjective interpretations; meanwhile, to a radical constructivist, there is, potentially, no external reality, or at least one we can access. As Anderson said, radical constructivists "regard reality as the construction of the mind, emphasizing the autonomy of the self and the individual as the meaning-maker" (1997, p. 43).

If you are perplexed, ask yourself the following questions:

1. How do I believe knowledge is constructed?
   a. *Constructivist:* I believe knowledge is constructed by individuals' mental processes based on their subjective experiences in an objective reality.
   b. *Radical constructivist:* I believe knowledge is constructed by individuals' mental processes, with no objective reality.
2. Do I believe there is an objective, external reality?
   a. *Constructivist:* Yes, an external reality exists independently from me.
   b. *Radical constructivist:* I am skeptical about it. (It may all be in my mind).

This complexity leads straight to social constructionism: a third, distinct epistemology essential to understanding postmodern family therapy. Anderson (1997) attributed the first stirrings of social constructionism in the social sciences to Berger and Luckmann as well as credited more recent contributors such as Bruner, Goodman, Gergen, Harré, Shotter, Polkinghorne, Sarbin, Geertz, and Taylor (pp. 40–41). She cited Ken Gergen's description of social constructionism as a process "by which people come to describe, explain, or otherwise account for the world (including themselves) in which they live" (as cited in 1997, p. 41). Alluding to Gergen, Anderson expanded on the epistemology: "Knowledge is a communal construction, a product of social exchange; the relationship is the locus of knowledge" (p. 41). It is essential to know that one cannot understand postmodern family therapy models such as C-DP, narrative therapy, or SFBT without an understanding of social constructionist philosophy.

If we revisit our earlier questions, we now have a third option.

1. How do I believe knowledge is constructed?
   a. *Constructivist:* I believe knowledge is constructed by individuals' mental processes based on their subjective experiences in an objective reality.
   b. *Radical constructivist:* I believe knowledge is constructed by individuals' mental processes, with no objective reality.
   c. *Social constructionist:* I think knowledge is constructed in communities, and socio-cultural factors play a role in shaping our knowledge.
2. Do I believe there is an objective, external reality?
   a. *Constructivist:* Yes, an external reality exists independently from me.
   b. *Radical constructivist:* I am skeptical about it. (It may all be in my mind).
   c. *Social constructionist:* I would not say one we can access, but it is not my focal point anyway. I am more interested in how culture and social processes shape our world.

Radical constructivism and social constructionism are both epistemologies that see the world as unknowable in any absolute sense. Where they differ is in the emphasis on the individual or the community. Radical constructivists assume the individual constructs knowledge and reality (1997, p. 23). Contrastingly, social constructionists, unsurprisingly, emphasize the social aspect and believe knowledge is constructed communally in societies. As social constructionist Ken Gergen said, "Social constructionism places the origin of knowledge in social process. For social constructionists, the categories are not 'in the head' but in our language" (2023, p. 40). While constructivism focuses on subjectivity and shares some similarities with postmodernism, radical constructivism and social constructionism are firmly rooted in the postmodern movement, which challenges norms and traditional societal notions associated with modernist ways of seeing the world.

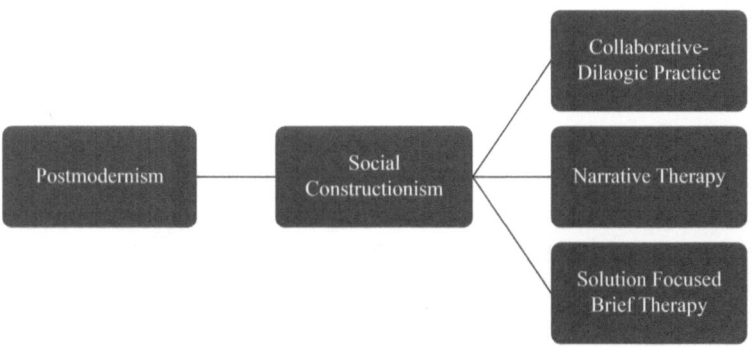

FIGURE 0.1 Postmodern, social constructionist family therapy models

Positivism, empiricism, and post-positivism

Positivism

A *positivist stance* is a modernist philosophical and scientific approach that aims to find Truth about our world through empirical observations. Positivism is often associated with quantitative research, which uses the scientific approach to look at objective data such as numerical data. A type of objective analysis is used, such as statistical analysis, to measure and quantify relationships and patterns. The epistemology underpinning positivism is that knowledge is empirically available to be found and investigated. Thus a positivist researcher almost always carries out their research via the scientific method, forming verifiable or falsifiable hypotheses. Positivism rejects claims that cannot be empirically tested, which is why quantitative researchers often strive to eliminate or minimize bias and researchers' emotions in their experiments.

Empiricism

Empiricism is an epistemological approach that closely aligns with positivism, arguing that knowledge, to be knowledge, must be rooted in verifiable data. Empiricists emphasize sensory data and observation as the vehicles of knowledge and grounds for Truth. Empiricists will use touch, taste, smell, sight, and hearing as data, believing that meticulous observation will establish verifiable results. An empiricist conviction is that first-hand experience is the foundation for objectivity and claims to veracity (Gergen, 2009). Positivism and empiricism are two forms of modernism. Sometimes, postmodernists will use these terms interchangeably, but it is important to note the subtle differences. To help clarify the differences between positivism and empiricism, consider this question:

1. What is the primary source of knowledge and truth in research?
    a. *Empiricist:* I believe knowledge and truth are obtained through objective facts verifiable by our five senses.
    b. *Positivist:* I believe knowledge and truth are obtained through systematic processes, predominantly the scientific method, involving observation, measurement, and strict adherence to methodologies to develop scientific theories.

Empiricism and positivism are both modernist.

Post-positivism

Now you are well on your way to understanding postmodernism in contrast to positivist and empiricist assumptions. *Post-positivism* is a skepticism of modernism. It falls under postmodern philosophy and is a stance that questions the assumptions positivists can take for granted. Examples include the modernist assumptions of an objective reality, universal laws, and absolute certainty. Modernist assumptions also include the idea that a person can be value-free, neutral, and/or devoid of personal biases; it assumes one can be an objective observer. Post-positivism challenges all those ideas.

Social constructionism, the key underpinning of the three postmodern models discussed in this book, is steeped in post-positivism. A social constructionist would adopt a post-positivist stance and look questioningly upon overlooked propositions. Post-positivism emphasizes the subjectivity of the researchers as well as what is researched, arguing that any objectivity is an illusion. Knowledge, language, and culture always influence our perspectives in how we construct even the categories we study; therefore, we create what we study rather than study what is "out there." The phrase "out there" implies objectivity. Post-positivists and social constructionists converge in their denial of the possibility of objective facts or an objective reality.

Consider the following research questions for yourself:

1. What do I believe is the goal of research?
   a. *Positivist:* I believe the goal is to discover objective, universal facts about the world.
   b. *Post-Positivist:* I believe the goal is to consider subjective experiences, meanings, and contexts.
2. What do I believe is the role of empirical evidence?
   a. *Positivist:* I believe empirical evidence establishes objective, measurable facts.
   b. *Post-Positivist:* I believe empirical evidence is influenced by subjectivity, which is embedded throughout every aspect of the research.
3. How do I view the nature of knowledge in research?
   a. *Positivist:* Knowledge is derived from our objective world.
   b. *Post-Positivist:* Knowledge is constructed through social processes within communities.

PERSPECTIVE VS. WORLDVIEW: MODERNIST LANGUAGE VS. POSTMODERNIST LANGUAGE

It is philosophically important to use the language of "worldview" rather than "perspective" when entering a postmodern space. Although this seems like "just semantics," the two words mean very different things in an epistemological context. *Worldview* is a postmodern term, while *perspective* has modernist roots.

Think of the famous allegory in which blind men are inspecting an elephant. In that example, one individual feels the trunk, one the tail, and so on. From a positivist lens, the elephant represents an objective reality that can be understood through empirical, methodological observation and testing, with every person's *perspective* culminating in a greater knowledge about the Real* elephant. Each has a different perspective on *the* thing—the elephant. However, this assumes the "God's eye view" of them getting a piece of *the* Truth. To use perspective is to imply that "events are happening out there, just as God would see them, irrespective of anyone's particular impression" (Gergen, 2023, p. 58).

Contrast this to speaking of someone's worldview. Speaking of an individual's worldview honors the client's relationship to their truths and reality. From a radical constructivist lens, each person constructs their individual *worldview*, making it valid in its own right. We do not have access to the Real elephant; therefore, radical constructivists do not know if there *really is* one elephant, many elephants, or no elephants.

Like radical constructivists, social constructionists do not make Truth-claims about the elephant, and the so-called facts depend on community agreement since there is no way to directly access the elephant. What modernists may call facts, social constructionists may call discourses, narratives, or stories. From this lens, the validity or nonvalidity is co-created between people. Gergen explained a social constructionist lens in research this way: "Researchers may enlighten each other, but the results will not converge" (2023, p. 78), and thus he cautioned readers to "beware of claims to objective truth" (2023, p. 78). Multiple worldviews, even contradictory worldviews, are permitted and often encouraged in a postmodern, social constructionist stance. If I can be reductive for the sake of introducing the concept, you might consider the differences between the phrases "find the truth" and "live your truth." Marinate on this for a bit. What are the implications of this shift in language on psychotherapeutic work?

Science wars

Again, empiricism and positivism belong to modernist philosophy; post-positivism crosses into postmodern philosophy. See Figure 0.2 below.

The tension between an empiricist/positivist and a post-positivist theory is palpable, culminating in hostile "science wars" in research and academia (Gergen, 2001). While debates still exist with researchers fighting over which theory is best or most useful, there is a current trend to highlight postmodernism as a different way of thinking, being, and viewing the world—rather than being purely oppositional to modernism.

While postmodernism critiques and challenges many modernist ideas, postmodernism is also more nuanced. Remember, postmodernism is a movement that reaches beyond therapy or research, such as art, literature, and architecture. We should be cautious about oversimplifying the relationship and characterizing it merely as confrontational. Present-day leaders in postmodern family therapy, such as Ken Gergen and Harlene Anderson, invite us to see postmodern practices as something to try on to see whether they fit for us (e.g., Gergen, 2023) rather than pull out the stakes and pitchforks.

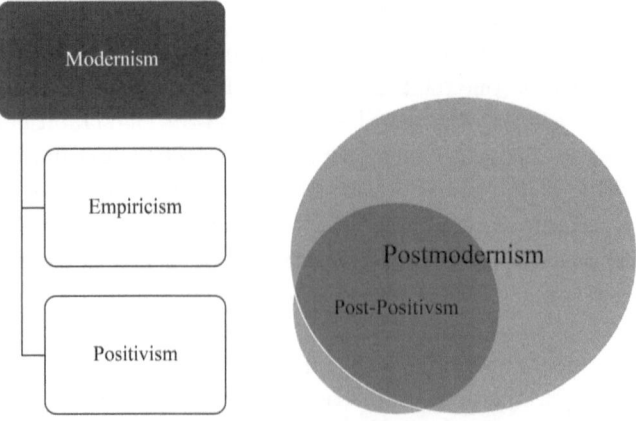

FIGURE 0.2 Empiricism, positivism, and post-positivism

Structuralism and post-structuralism

Structuralism is a movement that focuses on physical parts and their organization. It emphasizes the hierarchy and organization in institutions. General Systems Theory uses structuralist metaphors, especially to highlight the interconnectedness of parts of a system. *Post-structuralism* is a critical reaction to structuralism. It questions the presumed stability that structuralists postulate organizations have. Post-structuralism, heavily influenced by the philosopher Michel Foucault, does not see things as static. As SFBT founders Steve de Shazer and Insoo Kim Berg (1992) described, "For structuralists, meanings are stable and knowable through transformation, but for post-structuralists, meanings are seen as known through social interaction. Minimally, post-structuralists question the opposition of the subject and the object upon which the possibility of objectivity depends" (pp. 73–74). Let me summarize: structuralism falls under the modern umbrella, while post-structuralism falls under the postmodern umbrella. Thus structuralism proposes objective meanings, and post-structuralism challenges the idea of objective meanings and focuses instead on social interaction versus parts of a system. Breaking it down further, structuralism focuses on the building and corporate hierarchical structure (e.g., CEO, COO, CFO), and post-structuralism focuses on the people interacting within the building (i.e., communication dynamics). Instead of "top-down" or "bottom-up," post-structuralism is a horizontal approach. This applies in business as much as it does in therapy. The postmodern models (i.e., C-DP, narrative therapy, and SFBT) lean into post-structuralism over structuralism. You can see this in how those models navigate the hierarchy and power dynamics of therapist-client.

Comparing modern and postmodern models

Psychodynamic therapy, CBT, emotionally focused therapy, and the Gottman Method share a modernist philosophical foundation. Psychodynamic theory focuses on exploring the unconscious. CBT focuses on changing maladaptive thoughts and behaviors. Emotionally focused therapy focuses on attachment theory, and although it may have aspects of postmodern thought, it aligns closer to modernist views. The Gottman Method uses observational analysis, assessments, and skill building, making it staunchly modern.

Some modernist family therapy models are the MRI, Milan systemic therapy, structural family therapy, strategic family therapy, and Bowen family therapy. MRI focuses on interventions—"the difference that makes a difference." Milan systemic therapy focuses on interventions and disrupting dysfunctional patterns. Structural family therapy focuses on interventions, hierarchy, and directives. Strategic family therapy focuses on interventions and observable changes. Bowen family therapy focuses on intergenerational patterns in a family. You will notice that most modernist models are interventionist models. Although the modernist family therapy models can be systemic and relational, they are built on underlying modernist principles: assuming one reality, assuming you can get closer to Truth, and assuming you can uncover what is "really going on."

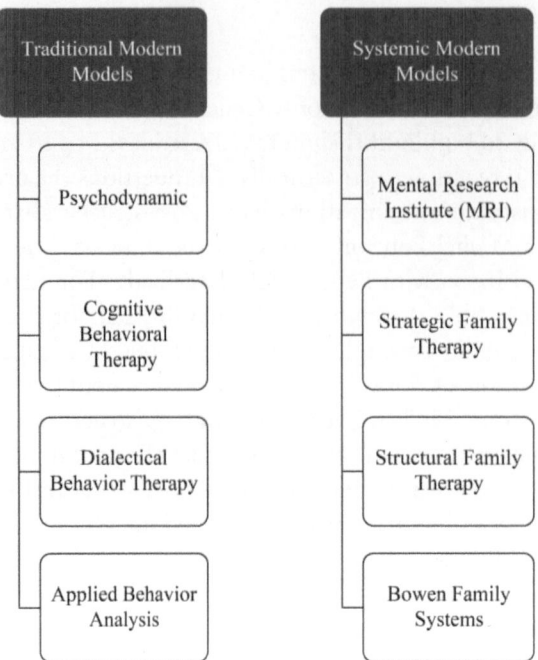

FIGURE 0.3 Comparing modern models

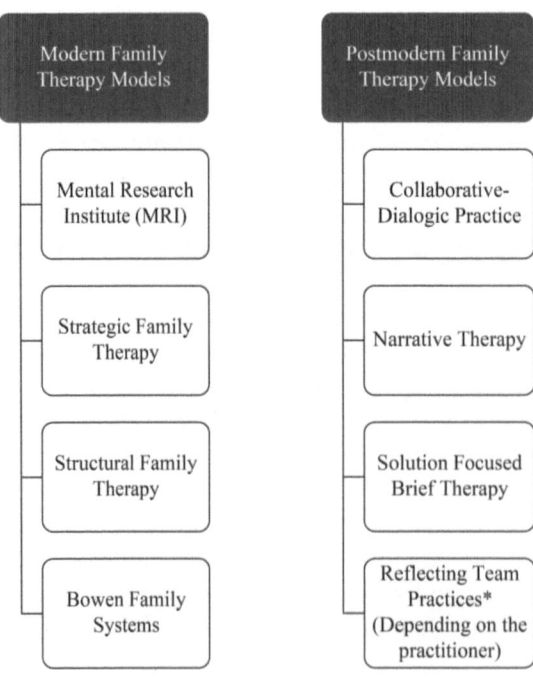

FIGURE 0.4 Comparing family therapy models

Of course, postmodern family therapy models came later, developing in keeping with the evolving times. Although it is now nearly 50 years old, postmodern family therapy is frequently described as "new." Certainly, "new" is relative to Freud's theory, introduced 125 years ago. But the description of postmodern ideas as new is misleading. Modernist practices are still widely used, and it is up to you to decide which philosophy mostly aligns with the practitioner you want to be and the values you hold.

SUMMARIZING EPISTEMOLOGICAL PARADIGMS

This section delved into different epistemological paradigms, focusing on modernism and postmodernism; constructivism, radical constructivism, and social constructionism; positivism, empiricism, and post-positivism. Modernism represents traditional and structured approaches. Postmodernism challenges established norms and embraces multiple worldviews.

Constructivism acknowledges an external reality filtered through subjective interpretations, emphasizing the role of individual mental schemas. Radical constructivism doubts the ability to access an independent reality, suggesting that all knowledge is a product of individual mental schemas. Social constructionism questions our access to an independent reality and views knowledge as a communal construction influenced by culture and social processes; meanwhile, a social constructionist epistemology emphasizes the relational construction of knowledge.

Positivism, a modernist philosophical approach, aims to discover objective truths through empirical observations and strict methodological research. Empiricism closely aligns with positivism, emphasizing sensory data and observation as the basis for knowledge. Post-positivism, a postmodern approach, questions positivist assumptions and emphasizes the subjectivity of researchers and their influence on knowledge. It is important to understand these paradigms as they play a significant role in shaping our ways of knowing what we (think we) know.

In family therapy literature, you may encounter post-positivism, post-structuralism, or social constructionism used interchangeably with postmodernism. By now, you understand that each one is an independent philosophy with its own implications. These are all different pieces that contribute to the larger puzzle.

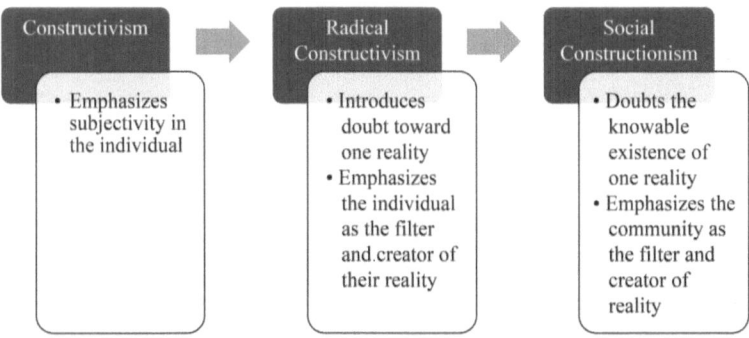

FIGURE 0.5 The chronological development toward social constructionism

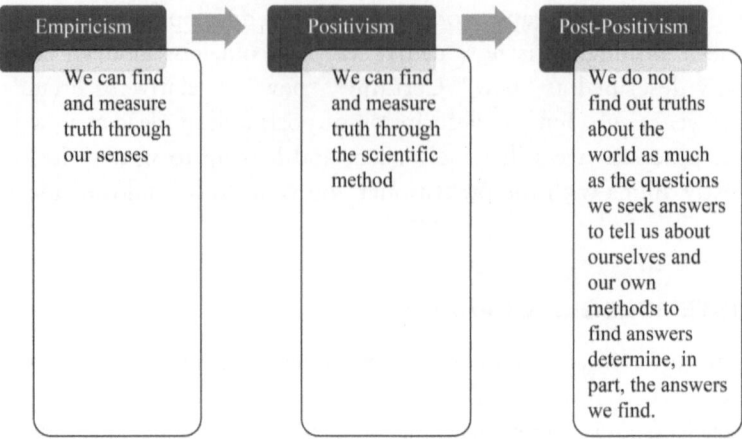

FIGURE 0.6 The chronological development toward post-positivism

REFLECTIVE QUESTIONS

1. Do you believe in an independent, external reality?
2. Do you believe we have access to it?
3. Do you believe knowledge is derived from this objective reality?
4. Do you believe personal experiences and interpretations shape knowledge?
5. Do you believe knowledge is influenced by culture, language, and norms?

Keywords

Modernism

Postmodernism

Social Constructionism

Constructivism

Radical Constructivism

Social Constructionism

Positivism

Empiricism

Post-Positivism

Perspective

Worldview

Epistemology

Ontology

Metaphysics

Structuralism

Post-Structuralism

Post-test*

*These are general answers; the specifics will depend on your model of choice.

1. What is the role of a therapist?
   a. *Modernist:* I believe the role of the therapist is to provide expert knowledge, directives, suggestions, or interventions.
   b. *Postmodernist:* I believe the role of the therapist is to collaboratively explore meanings and/or narratives.

2. What is the goal of a therapist?
   a. *Modernist:* I believe the goal of the therapist is to achieve concrete, often measurable outcomes and/or milestones.
   b. *Postmodernist:* I believe the goal of the therapist is to facilitate conversations around meanings and/or narratives.

3. How do you think change happens in therapy?
   a. *Modernist:* I believe therapeutic change happens through a change in patterns, behavior, literal thoughts, and/or perspective.
   b. *Postmodernist:* I believe therapeutic change happens through dialogue and often involves deconstructing limiting narratives and facilitating client empowerment through dialogue. This process creates new constructions of meanings, thoughts, and actions.

4. Should a therapist give advice?
   a. *Modernist:* I believe a therapist should give advice when appropriate.
   b. *Postmodernist:* I believe a therapist should generally replace advice with questions for clients to reflect upon and answer themselves.

5. How does a therapist find out what the problem is?
   a. *Modernist:* A therapist identifies problems through intake paperwork, assessments, observation, and clients' self-reports.
   b. *Postmodernist:* A therapist generally relies solely or primarily on clients' descriptions of what is a problem to them.

6. Should a therapist give homework?
   a. *Modernist:* Homework can sometimes be a helpful tool to enhance therapeutic outcomes.
   b. *Postmodernist:* I worry prescriptive homework may reinforce a more hierarchical therapeutic structure, but clients are welcome to do as they see fit.

7. What should a therapist do if a client fails to do their homework?
   a. *Modernist:* I believe the client is resistant to treatment and/or has another underlying barrier I want to explore.
   b. *Postmodernist:* I believe a therapist should not bring up homework unless the client does, and I would never label a client as "resistant."

8. Should therapists self-disclose information about themselves?
   a. *Modernist:* This should be avoided. A therapist should maintain professional distance and likely abstain from self-disclosure due to the dangers of boundary crossing.

b. *Postmodernist:* This is a matter of building discernment, not an automatic boundary viola-tion. A therapist's self-disclosure can enhance the depth of the therapeutic relationship, but it still needs to be done with care.

9. What should a therapist's treatment plan look like?

a. *Modernist:* A treatment plan needs specific, often measurable goals and objective indica-tions of progress.

b. *Postmodernist:* There is no objective indication of progress, so a treatment plan should have some inherent flexibility built in and be based on what the client believes is progress, not the therapist.

10. At what point is a client non-compliant?

a. *Modernist:* A client is non-compliant when they resist treatment and do not follow through with the treatment plan.

b. *Postmodernist:* "Non-compliance" is not a term I use or believe in, and we should not patholo-gize when a client does not do what we say or want them to do. We should be curious instead.

11. How close should a therapist be to their clients? How close is too close?

a. *Modernist:* Therapists can be supportive but with professional distance. You are too close if you become personally invested in client outcomes.

b. *Postmodernist:* Therapists should not be afraid of genuine human connection and ethical vulnerability; these are individuals interacting, after all. However, therapists need to follow ethical codes and abstain from friendships and certainly romantic relationships with clients.

12. What is the function of language in therapy?

a. *Modernist:* Language is a tool for communication.

b. *Postmodernist:* Language constructs our realities and can deconstruct unhelpful narratives.

13. Should a therapist use "we" language?

a. *Modernist:* In general, the use of "we" language is a "red flag" that the therapist is too close and should be used sparingly, if at all.

b. *Postmodernist:* Therapists may use "we" language to convey collaboration but always with an awareness of power dynamics and potential pitfalls. Discernment needs to be cultivated here as well.

14. When should a therapist terminate sessions?

a. *Modernist:* In general, sessions are terminated when treatment goals are met.

b. *Postmodernist:* In general, sessions are terminated when the client decides they no longer want or need sessions.

15. How does a therapist know whether therapy is successful?

a. *Modernist:* Success is measured by the client's ability to hit certain milestones and whether they achieved the treatment goals.

b. *Postmodernist:* Success is defined by the client; I should ask them if they found therapy helpful.

PRIMARY SOURCES

Anderson, H. (1997). *Conversation, language, and possibilities: A postmodern approach to therapy*. Basic Books.

Anderson, H. (2016). Postmodern/poststructural/social construction therapies: Collaborative, narrative, and solution-focused. In T. L. Sexton & J. Lebow (Ed.), *Handbook of family therapy: The science and practice of working with families and couples* (2nd dig. ed., pp. 182–204). Routledge.

Anderson, H. (2023). Conceptual framework: Emerging orienting sensitivities for relationships and conversations that invite transformation and possibility. In H. Anderson & D. R. Gehart (Eds.), *Collaborative-dialogic practice: Relationships and conversations that make a difference across contexts and cultures* (pp. 19–33, dig ed.). Routledge.

Anderson, H., & Burney, J. P. (1996). Collaborative inquiry: A postmodern approach to organizational consultation. *Human Systems: The Journal of Systemic Consultation and Management, 7*(2-3), 171–188.

Anderson, H., & Gehart, D. R. (Eds.). (2023). *Collaborative-dialogic practice: Relationships and conversations that make a difference across contexts and cultures* (dig. ed.). Routledge.

de Shazer, S. (1991). *Putting difference to work*. W. W. Norton & Company.

de Shazer, D., & Berg, I. K. (1992). Doing therapy: A post-structuralist re-vision. *Journal of Marital and Family Therapy, 18*(1), 71–81.

de Shazer, S., Dolan, Y., Korman, H., Trepper, T., McCollum, T., & Berg, I. K. (2021). *More than miracles: The state of the art of solution focused brief therapy* (Classic 2nd ed.). Routledge.

Gergen, K. J. (2001). *Social construction in context*. Sage.

Gergen, K. J. (2009). Social constructionist movement in modern psychology. *INTERthesis, 6*(1), 299–325.

Gergen, K. J. (2023). *An introduction to social construction: Co-creating the future* (4th dig. ed.). Sage.

Hoffman, L. (2001). *Family therapy: An intimate history* (dig. ed.). W. W. Norton.

White, M., & Epston, D. (1990). *Narrative means to therapeutic ends*. W. W. Norton.

Wittgenstein, L. (2009). *Philosophical investigations* (G. E. M. Anscombe, P. M. S. Hacker, & J. Schulte Trans., rev. 4th dig. ed.). Wiley Blackwell. (Original work published 1953).

Additional References

Bannink, F. P. (2007). Solution focused brief therapy. *Journal of Contemporary Psychotherapy, 37*, 87–94.

Cairns, D. (2015). Ψυχή, Θυμός, and metaphor in Homer and Plato. *Études Platoniciennes*. https://doi.org/10.4000/etudesplatoniciennes.566

Chang, C.-h. (2017). Compare differences between different Bible translations in the view of globalization: Illustrated by the case of "ψυχη" in the new testament. *Cultural and Religious Studies, 5*(10), 622–638.

Chenail, R. J., Reiter, M. D., Torres-Gregory, M., & Ilic, D. (2020). Postmodern family therapy. *The Handbook of Systemic Family Therapy, 1*, 417–442.

Ilic, D. (2017). *Conversation analysis of Michael White's decentered and influential position*. Nova Southeastern University. https://nsuworks.nova.edu/shss_dft_etd/25.

Mark, J. A. (2018). *The Egyptian afterlife & the feather of truth*. World History Encyclopedia. https://www.worldhistory.org/article/42/the-egyptian-afterlife–the-feather-of-truth/

Sartwell, C. (2013, June 19). Andy Warhol and the persistence of modernism. *New York Times Opinionator*. https://authenticationinart.org/pdf/artmarket/20130619-Andy-Warhol-and-the-Persistence-of-Modernism-NYT.pdf

PART II

Collaborative-Dialogic Practice (Formerly Collaborative Therapy)

CHAPTER 1

An introduction to collaborative-dialogic practice

....

Remember, as you read through these chapters, you can always return to the Introduction to refresh your memory on the terms you learned such as epistemology, ontology, post-positivism, and social constructionism.

QUESTIONS TO THINK ABOUT

1. How did collaborative-dialogic practice (C-DP) come to be founded, and where does it fit historically in family therapy?
2. Is there a difference between doing therapy collaboratively and working from a collaborative-dialogic (C-D) stance?
3. How is C-DP a confluence of hermeneutics and social constructionism?
4. Why are goals and the role of the therapist so different in this approach?
5. What role does philosophy play in C-DP?

According to Anderson's statements in an interview with Tapio Malinen (2004), Harlene Anderson joined a group in Galveston, Texas, called "Multiple Impact Therapy," which shared similarities to family therapy. Twenty years earlier, Harold (Harry) Goolishian had joined the same group. These like-minded psychology scholars connected, and together, they co-founded a model they called "collaborative language systems" (CLS). In 1997, Anderson described their model in depth in her seminal work entitled *Conversation, Language, and Possibilities: A Postmodern Approach to Therapy.* Over time, her model came to be known as *"collaborative therapy"* and most recently as *"collaborative-dialogic practice"* (C-DP) (see Anderson & Gehart, 2023).

DOI: 10.4324/9781003439349-3

When brainstorming about what the name of the model should be, Anderson and Goolishian wanted to call their approach something that emphasized the relationship between the client and therapist; words like cooperative and collaborative came to mind. Finding that collaborative and cooperative had very similar definitions in the dictionary, they chose "collaborative" in a bit of a "coin flip" but overall found that "collaborative" emphasized the more-egalitarian-than-not rapport that is built between therapist and client during the process of therapy (Hoff & Anderson, 2016). In other words, the therapist will speak with the client as more of a partner than a teacher or expert.

Anderson and Goolishian focused on *language* as a constructive system as opposed to previous marriage and family therapy predecessors that employed general systems and cybernetic ways of thinking, which presupposed that the symptom served a function in the family system (Haley, 2010). Anderson and Goolishian were not interested in the physical constructs of a system but in how language constructs a system.

As opposed to what original family therapists practiced—from what Goolishian called an "onion theory" perspective (Anderson, 1997): "Like the core of an onion, surrounded by outer layers, the individual is encircled by the family, the family by the larger system, the larger system by the community, and so forth" (p. 19), Anderson and Goolishian differentiated their model as a *language systems theory* model (1988). The onion theory presumes a symptom has a function in the family, school, place of worship, or a larger system. In contrast, a language system theory presupposes that language is creating the system rather than the system pre-existing.

This is why *social constructionism* is so fundamental to Anderson and Goolishian's now-named model, *collaborative-dialogic practice* (C-DP). *Social constructionism* is the belief that language creates reality. As you will recall from the Introduction, this therapist is more interested in an individual's truth and reality than the "One Truth" and "One Reality."

Anderson (2012a) left the language systems theory metaphor behind, saying that there are other metaphors that better describe the therapeutic practice.

> As predicted when Harry Goolishian and I concluded our 1988 article "Human Systems as Linguistic Systems," what seemed like plausible ideas then have evolved over time. At that time, we were immersed in exploring a language systems metaphor for our work and had left behind mechanical cybernetic systems metaphors. No longer thinking of human systems as social systems defined by social organization, we viewed them as language systems distinguished by

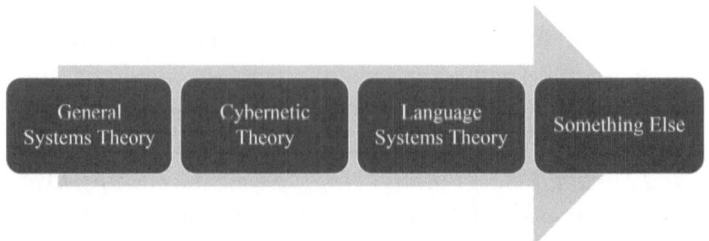

FIGURE 1.1 Harlene Anderson and Harry Goolishian's trajectory and chronological progression

respective linguistic and communicative markers. *Since then,* the language systems metaphor, although important, has faded into the background as I continued to explore other organizing metaphors for my practice experiences.

(p. 8, italics added for emphasis)

THE HISTORICAL EVOLUTION OF COLLABORATIVE-DIALOGIC PRACTICE (C-DP)

Over the years, co-founders Anderson and Goolishian were consistently fascinated by language. Like many family therapists, Anderson and Goolishian were initially drawn in by the *general systems theory* and *cybernetic theory* work of the Mental Research Institute (MRI) founded by Gregory Bateson, Don Jackson, John Weakland, and Jay Haley (Anderson, 1997). They were intrigued by MRI's focus on the family system instead of one dysfunctional individual (Anderson & Goolishian, 1991) as well as their strategic use of language (Anderson, 2012b) to create change through "therapists' ideas, comments, questions, interventions, and homework assignments" (Malinen, 2004, pp. 68–69).

Next, Anderson and Goolishian were introduced to the *constructivist* work of Maturana and Valera, which led them to view language differently: as a constructive, not instructive, process of interaction (Anderson, 1997, 2023a; Anderson & Goolishian, 1991). Anderson and Goolishian also discovered the philosophy of *hermeneutics*: the "interpretation of interpretations" (1991, p. 22), which included Heidegger's, then Gadamer's, then Habermas' study of the interpretation of language (Anderson, 1997). Anderson and Goolishian seemed to resonate with Heidegger's focus on *being-in-the-world* and recursivity. Their investigations outside of family therapy led them to other diverse philosophers such as Wittgenstein, Vygotsky, Bakhtin, and Derrida (as well as novelist Dostoyevsky), whose works centered around the use of language, the meaning of language, and the plurality of voices in discourse (Anderson, 1997; Anderson & Gehart, 2007). Undoubtedly, this is not an exhaustive list of philosophers who struck a chord with C-DP's founders.

As addressed later, Anderson found the most resonance with contemporary philosophers Ken Gergen and John Shotter, whose *social constructionist* ideas underlie Anderson's approach (Anderson, 2007b; Hoff & Anderson). Illustratively, Anderson and Goolishian summarized the confluence of hermeneutics and social constructionism (1991) as a "postmodern shift where one cannot have direct knowledge of the world because what is known is not independent of the person; it is the product of interactions between persons" (p. 22). While social constructionism is the foremost philosophical pillar, each of the aforementioned philosophers ignited Anderson and Goolishian's interest in language and reality, contributing to the development of C-DP (Anderson, 2007d).

A PHILOSOPHICAL STANCE, NOT A MODEL

Although Anderson came from a background in psychology (Hoff & Anderson), she found herself delving into philosophy—especially *epistemological* and *ontological* philosophy—with her mentor Goolishian, explaining, "That's where the language seemed to be that helped us better understand and describe our experiences and what clients were telling us about their experiences of therapy" (Malinen, pp. 68–69). As Anderson stated in her first book and reiterated throughout her career, her collaborative approach is *more of a philosophy* than a theory or model (e.g., Anderson, 1997, 2001). She explained her reasoning: philosophers have long focused on the human experience and what it means to be human (Anderson, 2001), including "self-identity, agency, mind, relationships, and futures; meanwhile, *theory* informs methods by creating types and categories of people" (Anderson & Gehart, 2007, p. xix, italics added for emphasis) and can be limiting and "myopic" (Anderson, 2007e, p. 43).

Anderson and Goolishian rebelled against the generalization of people and the universalization of their problems via methods and theories. Instead of the dominant psychotherapeutic practice of treating individuals as types of people, Anderson's philosophical stance encourages mutual curiosity and hesitation towards labeling or cataloging individuals (Gergen et al., 1996). Anderson's approach is built upon unique relationships and conversations with clients wherein each client is fully humanized and treated as a distinct individual with a distinct set of problems or circumstances (Anderson, 2014, 2023b). C-DP challenges an absolute position that there are "kinds of people" or people with "kinds of problems."

This philosophical stance is not part of a therapeutic theory, method, or formula. It is relationally oriented and authentic to the person operating from it. Anderson said, "Philosophy is not about finding scientific truths" (Anderson, 2001, p. 347). She later elaborated: "Philosophy involves ongoing analysis, inquiry, and reflection with self and others. It is not about finding truths, scientific or otherwise, nor is it about objects or things; it is about people (Anderson, 2007e, p. 43).

Instead of "model," Anderson preferred the word "stance" "because it is a way of being internally as a person and externally with others" (Anderson, 1996, p. 200). A therapist practicing from this stance embodies certain beliefs that govern and orient the session. There is no recipe to follow in C-DP. Anderson's philosophical stance is a thoughtful, nonformulaic position that is inherently respectful and appreciative of human differences.

The therapist practicing from this philosophical stance ensures clients know they "have something to say that is worthy of hearing" (Anderson, 2007f, p. 4). C-D practitioners hold space for interconnectedness between linguistics and ontology, and every therapist-client relationship is approached differently (Anderson, 2007e). Because of this, Anderson said it was often easier to demonstrate C-DP than explain it (e.g., Anderson, 2023a). During a C-D session, questions and comments arise naturally for both the client and therapist through what Lynn Hoffman called "contagious curiosity" (Hoff & Anderson).

MOVING ON FROM MRI AND CYBERNETIC THEORY

Feeling cybernetic family therapy models were perhaps overly structured, strategic, calculated, and directive, Anderson and Goolishian became less comfortable with the expert stance behind MRI and their contemporary family therapy models (Anderson, 1997; Hoff & Anderson; Malinen). For example, an MRI therapist might use a strategic, paradoxical intervention called "prescribing the symptom" in which the therapist addresses a couple's presenting problem of conflicts over household chores by directing one partner to neglect certain tasks like washing the dishes or doing laundry. The therapist's intent would be to disrupt the established pattern, prompting the partners to work together to create a more balanced division of household responsibilities and change their couple dynamic. Meanwhile, Anderson and Goolishian preferred a more straightforward approach that prioritized meaning and conversational connection over MRI's directive interventions (Anderson, 1997).

Anderson and Goolishian moved away from cybernetic and systems metaphors (Anderson, 2012a, 2012b; Malinen, 2004). Anderson and Goolishian became interested in the constructive nature of language and saw people as *"meaning-generating beings* as opposed to information-processing machines" (Anderson & Goolishian, 1992, p. 26). They began to see systems constructed by language, not systems organized by structure, and, as previously stated, they predominantly utilized a language systems metaphor until Anderson discovered other metaphors that were a better fit (Anderson, 2012a). For these reasons, neither "system" nor "structure" are words that do justice to C-DP, given the meanings those words carry over from cybernetic family therapy models (Malinen). Therefore, to focus on homeostasis, boundaries, family hierarchy, or intergenerational patterns or to see any necessary steps, sequences, techniques, or procedures would be to look at C-DP through a modernist lens. C-DP's shift aligned with other family therapy practitioners, including Tom Andersen (spelled with an "e") and Lynn Hoffman.

A PARADIGMATIC SHIFT

Social constructionist John Shotter and family therapists Lynn Hoffman, Tom Andersen, and Harlene Anderson were all inspired by *"withness,"* which can be cursorily described as "a process of orienting and re-orienting oneself to the other" (Anderson, 2012a, p. 13). Attributing the origin of this word to the philosopher Mikhail Bakhtin (pronounced "Mee-khah-eel Bahk-teen"), Anderson suggested *"withness"* may be even more helpful than "collaborative" in terms of helping others understand what she does in therapy (Hoff & Anderson).

Withness can be easy to do but difficult to explain. As part of the contextual development of C-DP's use of *withness* within family therapy, I review (1) reflecting team practices or reflecting processes (Anderson, 2007a; Shotter, 2007), (2) the use of *"both/ and"* language and thinking (Andersen, 2012), and (3) *withness* practices (Hoffman, 2007). *Withness* practice focuses on the human-to-human relationship in psychotherapy, a prominent feature in dialogic practices (Sidis et al., 2022). I like to call it "humans human-ing."

Reflecting team practices

Reflecting teams developed out of the Milan family therapy process, where a team of therapists would sit behind a one-way mirror and observe a therapist interacting with a family. Behind the mirror, the Milan team would converge to develop expert hypotheses about the family. They would then develop an intervention that would be shared with the family.

In contrast, Tom Andersen's team in Norway would invite the family members to listen directly to the therapists' thoughts, questions, and hypotheses. Generally, the team is listening to the family's thoughts, and this turned the tables such that the family was listening to the team's thoughts—as if peaking behind the curtain. This eliminated the need for musings about what therapists were surreptitiously discussing or writing down on their clipboards.

Reflecting teams invited the family to reflect upon the therapists' thoughts about their situation. Tom Andersen's reflecting process gave clients the chance to decide for themselves what was pertinent. The spirit of reflecting team practices is one of transparency, a lowered hierarchy, and "in-there-togetherness" (Anderson, 2007e; Anderson & Goolishian, 1991).

Harlene Anderson said this of reflecting team practices in postmodern family therapy: "Reflecting teams began a process of dialogues about dialogues that enabled new conversations, giving time and space for speaking and listening to the unspoken, and giving family members the choice to respond and how to respond" (Anderson & Jenson, 2007, p. xxi). The "unspoken" here refers to the hermeneutic-based ideas of the "said" and the "not-said-yet" (Anderson, 2007d), which emphasizes the creation of meaning through dialogue. Goolishian captured this idea when he said: "I never know what I mean until I say it" (as cited in Gehart et al., 2007, p. 373).

The "both/and"

Sometimes, Tom Andersen and his team noticed families reacting with what modernist psychotherapists would call "resistance" when they asked families if they had considered doing "x" instead of "y." Andersen would not conceptualize it in this way but rather put the burden of responsibility back on the therapist to listen more attentively and speak in a way that better fit with the client. Tom Andersen and his team altered their "either/or" language, noticing a remarkable change when they tweaked their wording to say to "both/and" language such as, "In addition to what you have been doing, could you also consider doing this?" (Andersen, 2012, p. 20). Not only was the therapists' use of *both/and* language a change in communication but, as Andersen himself stated, it was a "big philosophical and ideological change" (p. 20)—a change in the therapists' outlook. *Both/and language* evolved to *both/and thinking*, as opposed to *either/or thinking* (Shotter, 2007).

Since its introduction in the 1980s, Tom Andersen's *both/and* concept has become a well-known family therapy idea across models (Anderson, 2012b). It introduces curiosity through tentative language. This makes room for a plurality of voices, descriptions, and suggestions. The therapists' voices do not reign but can reverberate when clients find resonance with the therapists' multi-voiced, often-varied ideas.

Withness

Harlene Anderson, Lynn Hoffman, and Tom Andersen all practiced *withness*, which emphasizes the therapist's presence with clients, "including ways of thinking *with*, talking *with*, acting *with*, and responding *with* them" (Anderson, 2007f, p. 4). *Withness* is a way of really focusing in on the client's language, including verbal and nonverbal language (Anderson, 2012b, 2023a). It is a philosophical, co-creative process—not a technique—and *withness* practice is distinct from "aboutness" (Hoffman). Anderson clarified this difference as talking *with* clients (Anderson, 2007a, 2007b) rather than "to, for, at, or *about* them" (Hoff & Anderson, 14:46). There are no pre-planned thoughts and questions because the therapist is listening to the language with *in-the-moment* spontaneity.

Presence is key to *withness*, and the relational experience of being with the client is prioritized. The therapist pays attention not only to what the client is saying but also to the tone of the client's voice, gesticulations, and expressions on their face. Contrast this to listening for an opportunity to ask the so-called right questions. Tom Andersen described *withness* practice as "to just see, hear, feel, and *not think*" (Andersen, 2012, p. 21).

In an interview, Harlene Anderson and Tapio Malinen discussed this as a dialogical shift away from giving directives, trying to sway clients' opinions, or offering plans to alter behaviors. C-DP's approach is one of conversationally *wandering* with clients (Malinen). As further explained in her book with Gehart, Anderson said: "Like walking hand in hand through a forest at night without a flashlight, we are jointly feeling, exploring our way forward" (Anderson, 2023b, p. 39).

This *withness*-wandering with others is at the heart of C-DP and, as Shotter said, is a "dynamic" participatory process (Anderson, 2007e, p. 45). It requires therapists to interact earnestly with clients. The essence lies in exploring the complexities of each client's experience. This includes not labeling them under psychotherapeutic categories, as most of us are taught to do (Anderson, 1997; Gergen et al., 1996; Hoff & Anderson).

A WAY TO EXPLAIN *WITHNESS*: RECIPROCITY, REFLEXIVITY, AND RECURSIVITY

In order to elaborate on *withness*, I address different ways of humans *being* with one another. *Withness* is a very human interaction where each person is open while also offering. The openness is seen, held, appreciated, and returned. Metaphoric language may capture this experience better than technical language. One person welcomes the other with open arms, an open mind, and an open heart. The other does the same, making this *reciprocal*.

Yet "reciprocal" does not fully capture the experience because reciprocity is often conceptualized linearly as a transactional exchange. A more advanced understanding is to see this interaction as *reflexive*. This highlights a more cyclical interaction where each human is informed by and continually informs the other. For new learners, a reflexive interaction can be thought of as a loop; meanwhile, an even more advanced understanding is to see this more aptly characterized as a dance.

> Sometimes a shade crosses the talker's face, the hands are closed or opened, there comes a cough, a tear can appear, or the person pauses. The listener understands that the spoken words carry a meaning that makes the talker re-experience something she has experienced before without understanding what that is. Often, the listener is carried away and moved by noticing that the talker is moved.
>
> *(Andersen, 2007, p. 92)*

Whereas the words "loop" or "cycle" have undercurrents of permanence or concretized causality, a "dance" emphasizes the continually evolving nature of the interaction.

Mutual reflexivity takes what has come before as it informs the present, which informs the future, which informs how the past is reinterpreted, which informs ... and so on. As Anderson and Goolishian (1991) said, "The generation of meaning is endless" (p. 32). Thus *withness* is an improvisational, reflexive process where each person is shaped and reshaped, and *touched* by the other (Anderson, 2007e).

If "reflexive" is a good description of the *withness* interaction between people, "recursive" is a good description of the conversation itself. While this also has hermeneutic (i.e., related to interpretation and the shaping and reshaping of meanings) connotations of a loop falling back upon itself, the emphasis moves from individuals to dialogue. In C-DP, the dialogue almost becomes an entity in itself as the therapist and client take part in its construction, development, and redevelopment with each turn in conversation (Anderson, 2023a, p. 26).

C-DP is both a reflexive and recursive process. *Anderson reinforced this when she said, "In the telling and retelling, not only do new stories emerge, but a person changes in relationship to them" (Anderson, 1997, p. 108).* The process (not content) of human interaction is emphasized. The dialogical activity is certainly greater than the sum of its parts, and something new emerges from the process. It is constantly evolving. Try to avoid a linear (i.e., cause → effect) conceptualization. More than an outcome, it is a profound, interminable meaning-making process where the past influences the present, which influences the future, which allows reflection on the past, which influences a new present understanding, which ... and so on (Anderson, 2007e). See Figure 1.2 for a comparison between reciprocity, reflexivity, and recursivity. A final word on reciprocity,

A. The Interaction of Being in Conversation

Reciprocity	Basic Understanding of Reflexivity	Advanced Understanding of Reflexivity
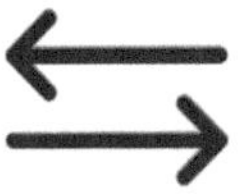	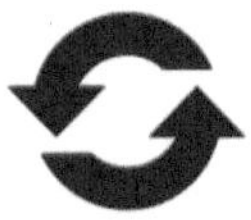	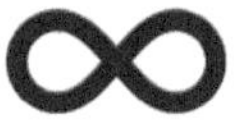
The activity of being in conversation is conceptualized linearly.	The activity of being in dialogical conversation is reflexive.	The activity of being in dialogical conversation is reflexive.

B. The Conversation Itself

Reciprocity	Basic Understanding of Recursivity	Advanced Understanding of Recursivity
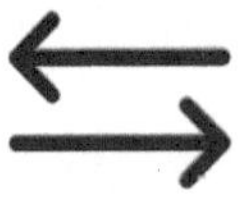	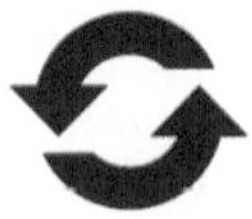	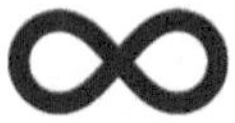
The dialogue itself is broken into parts of speaker and respondent.	The dialogue itself is whole and recursive.	The dialogue itself is whole and recursive.

FIGURE 1.2 An interactional and dialogical shift in conversations

reflexivity, and recursivity: they are often used by professionals interchangeably—especially the latter two—when trying to explain the intricacies of *withness*.

Sometimes, professional language can make what is clear seem cloudy, making us forget what we already know from our human experience. There is a difference between being physically present and being emotionally present. Furthermore, there is a spectrum of how emotionally present and vulnerable a person can be. Remember, there is a difference between having a conversation and having a conversation that *moves you*.

A comparison is sometimes made between Harlene Anderson's C-DP and Carl Rogers' person-centered therapy. Anderson addressed the similarities and differences between C-DP and person-centered therapy in an article in 2001. Some of the differences Anderson listed are Rogers' (1) causal, "if-then" thinking, (2) his interest in the "core self," and (3) his goal of "personality change" resulting from unconditional positive regard (pp. 342–349). A key difference Anderson underscored is her natural, authentic stance in her work which is beyond a posture and beyond a technique. We explore the specifics of her stance later in this chapter.

SHIFT IN THE ROLE OF THE THERAPIST

As Anderson and Goolishian began implementing collaborative work, the role of the therapist moved from modernist psychotherapeutic practices as an outside observer, examiner, detective (or, at worst, interrogator), and arbiter of right and wrong thoughts, behaviors, patterns, or family structures to something new (Anderson, 1997, 2007e). In C-DP, a therapist does not generalize, pathologize, use a toolkit, or follow a recipe. As a therapist, you do not fix clients because they are not broken. As Anderson said:

> I am often asked, for instance, "How do you treat child abuse?" or, "How do you work with eating disorders? Implicit in such questions is the assumption that there are across-the-board commonalities among problems. This paradigmatic shift in thinking can be jarring to therapists who believe that the target of treatment is a system defined by social theory (individual, couple, family, group) and that treatment repairs the defect (known pathological feature).
>
> *(1997, p. 77)*

Anderson's approach is not deficit-focused, nor does it cast broad generalizations upon people.

Mutual puzzling

In this new paradigmatic context, the therapist engages in *mutual puzzling*, pondering big questions with clients instead of (1) presuming to know what the problem "really" is, and/or (2) trying to convince clients to see what is "really" going on in the individual, couple, or family (Anderson, 1997). *Withness* is inherent in the mutual puzzling process. Anderson described this as a mutual inquiry (2007c, 2007e). One person's thoughts influence the other's, and so on. Hopefully, it is now clear that there is cooperation, alliance, and humanization in this process.

Anecdotally, I have noticed C-D practitioners tend to use their clients' names more frequently than modernist-practicing psychotherapists. Likewise, the clients more

TABLE 1.1 That sounds really hard

Modernist: Traditional Student-Therapist

Judith: That sounds really hard. Have you ...?

Client: Yes, I have tried that and x and y and z, and nothing works.

Judith: Well, did you ...?

Client: I know, I know, I should have done that, but I ....

Judith may have unintentionally created an environment of shame or failure. Her attempts to "fix it" may lead to her client feeling "stupid," incompetent, or otherwise lacking. Sometimes our attempts to find solutions for the person's problem (note: not necessarily the person, but the category of person) can leave clients feeling discouraged.

Postmodernist: Collaborative-Dialogic Student-Therapist

Judith: "That sounds really hard, Harry."

Client: "Thank you, Judith."

Judith created space for both parties to soak in the words, to feel the words' impact. Judith has no hidden agenda to jump to, and she can wait. Silence, screams, or sobs—all experiences are welcome. Nothing needs to be rushed; no boxes need to be ticked off. They both can just be. Together.

frequently use the name of the therapist. In my experience as a supervisor, it is not uncommon for me to hear a traditional therapist say something along the lines of, "That sounds really hard. Have you ...?" Concurrently, I witness my C-D therapists reacting with something like, "That sounds really hard, Harry." In response to the first, the client often says something along the lines of, "Yes, I have tried that and x and y and z, and nothing works" or, "I know, I know, I should have done that, but I .... " In response to the second way, the client may simply say, "Thank you, Judith." The therapist has room to respond with silence, waiting to see where the client may prefer to go next. I use this example to simply illustrate that the same words can land very differently depending on the therapist's underlying epistemological paradigm.

Let us look toward the table to notice differences between two versions of a session. There are, of course, many more complexities, but let us use a reductive example for learning the basics. Again, try to avoid jumping to a linear conceptualization that this exchange is about a technique or proper incorporation of micro-skills. Think of the process of the human-to-human interaction, not your preconceived ideas of what therapists "should" do. Imagine being in the room (or virtual room). How do you imagine you might feel if you were Harry or if you were Judith?

THE ROLE OF THE COLLABORATIVE-DIALOGIC THERAPIST

"Is there a difference between a dinner conversation with a good friend and a therapy conversation with a stranger?"

—*Harlene Anderson*

Anderson first posed this question in her seminal work, *Conversation, Language, and Possibilities: A Postmodern Approach to Therapy* (Anderson, 1997, p. 1). Your response will reveal your epistemology and inform the way you think about therapy and the therapeutic process. For Anderson, a C-D practitioner's role is to be a genuine listener and speaker who engages with clients in an "(inter)active" (Anderson, 2007f, p. 4) process. Since it is a philosophical position and attitude one takes on as a way of being, a therapist cannot be taught how to "do" C-DP per se (Anderson, 2007a, 2007e).

If you work from this stance, you understand that C-D therapeutic work is an ever-evolving partnership between client and therapist. The role of a postmodernist therapist here will not look the same as it would look in modernist family therapy. As Anderson, Goolishian, and Windermand said, "The role of the therapist is simply to engage in conversation" (1986, p. 10). However, presumably to make it easier for others to learn, Anderson adopted different metaphors to describe the process, such as having good manners and being polite as a host and guest (e.g., Anderson, 2012a, 2012b).

Be a polite host-guest

Anderson (1997, 2012b) used a *host-guest* metaphor wherein the therapist is a host, providing a safe space for clients while also being a guest in clients' lives. As a host, you greet people warmly and facilitate amiable dialogue. There are social subtleties too—perhaps a handshake, hug, or glance—that the host offers to help the guests feel more at ease. These often-unaddressed exchanges are unique every time, as the host and guests adapt moment-to-moment (Anderson, 2007e; Gehart, 2023). In a successful host-guest relationship, the host is likely to care about the comfort of the guest and, more often than not, assume the best of their guest's intentions. Perhaps it is helpful to think of the complex character relationship in French writer-philosopher Albert Camus' 1986 (pronounced "ka-moo") short story titled "L'Hôte." This French word means both "host" and "guest." Not only do you want to be a polite host, but you also want to be a gracious guest in their life who is invited back into later conversations (Hoff & Anderson).

A polite host would be unlikely to think their guest was "difficult," "resistant," or "unmotivated" (Anderson, 1984) if they were not fully engaged in the conversation or did not agree with the host. By being polite, the host would ask gentle questions, curious to know more about their guest's thoughts and make sense of their guest's actions. Additionally, they would likely take time to consider how they—as a host—might have contributed to any social disruption that may have occurred.

Note the contrast to higher education and professional mental health tendencies to view the client as the problem within supervision, consultations, or a therapist's private thoughts. When therapists hypothesize or reflect upon a client in the client's absence, they are still participating in the construction of a story about who the client *is,* which "suppresses the client's narrative" (Gergen, Hoffman, & Anderson, p. 5). Because C-DP psychotherapists acknowledge the relational component to constructing meaning, they remain aware of *how* they speak about their clients and to whom (as each partner in dialogue shapes meaning). It would be impolite to speak poorly about clients in their absence, and it would also have a lasting impact on how clinicians view their clients and make sense of their stories (see Malinen).

Cultivate genuine curiosity

Is there room for doubt or suspicion of psychotherapeutic knowledge we inherited in graduate school (Hoff & Anderson), work environments, and social media—or are we simply accepting of inherited knowledge that an individual is "a noncompliant patient," "resistant to treatment," or "a treatment failure?" In postmodernism, we must be skeptical of sweeping generalizations and grand narratives (Anderson, 2007f); moreover, in social constructionism, we must be cautious about our language—and others'—forming our realities (Anderson, 1997).

To adopt a C-D approach is to adopt a tentative, curious stance which lets the client inform you about who *they* think they are and what problems *they* identify (Anderson, 2007e, 2012a). From this position, not speaking poorly about your clients is not a mere procedure. The C-D therapist believes that language constructs reality, so they are cautious about who is involved in dialogue around "the problem." When therapists adopt this C-DP stance, they begin to genuinely see their clients differently—more as people experiencing life than as clients who are deficient in skill or limited by whatever someone has deemed is "wrong" with them.

Because of the inherent authenticity in this model, curiosity is an activity between individuals, not a technique performed by a therapist. The C-DP relationship plays a larger role, or at least a very different role, than it does in other modernist psychotherapeutic models. It may be helpful to consider the relationship itself to be the collaborative aspect, and the conversation itself to be the dialogical aspect—although this is an oversimplification that would leave us staunchly in modernist territory. Drawing distinct boundaries like I just did regresses to modernist black/white (i.e., either/or) thinking, which is antithetical to postmodern practices which are colloquially described as gray. Yet "gray" may be too bland to fit with the unending curiosity in this postmodern approach. Anderson's philosophy embraces a fuller kaleidoscope of meaning, one where meaning is always fluid and evolving. Contradictions are not only allowed but embraced.

> There was no such thing, therefore, as "a" problem, "a" solution, or even "a" family for that matter. There were at least as many descriptions of these as there were system members (including non-family system members). We were fascinated by these differences in language, especially the distinctions in descriptions, explanations, and meanings attributed to the same event or person. We sensed that somehow these differences were valuable and held possibilities, thought at the time we did not know in what way. We gave up trying to negotiate or blur differences or strive for consensus and instead let them be.
>
> *(Anderson, 2007c, p. 25)*

As you begin to practice C-DP, lead with your natural curiosity about who the client is and what sense *they* make of their lives, including the presenting problem and the people who contribute to the idea that "x" is a problem in the first place. Bringing us back to the Introduction, be curious about *their* worldview rather than impose your own. Clients' conceptualizations, hypotheses, and stories are prioritized; therefore, the therapist learns from the clients. It is an active process where "there is no room for boredom" (Anderson, 2001, p. 353). Therapists are encouraged to "try to respond in a way that relates to what the client is saying—not what they think the client should be saying" (Anderson, 2007f, p. 5).

Become a "conversational partner"

As a C-D practitioner, you want to be aware of your influence in the interpretation of truths and the construction of meaning. As befitting of a C-D therapist's *way of being* (Anderson, 2007e), the therapist is a *conversational partner* with clients in therapy, conversing dialogically and relating reflexively—just as they could with a mentor, friend, or family member. Thus Anderson said this position mirrors friendship, engaging in "telling, inquiring, interpreting, and shaping narratives" (1997, p. 95), yet the therapist certainly follows ethical codes and does not confuse clients for friends.

The two (or more) conversational partners take turns leading and following. Each has something to contribute to the conversation, and these contributions organically build upon one another, cumulatively forming and informing something new—a recursive dialogue. "As we become conversational partners with our client, the dialogue brings forth new ways of thinking and acting regarding dilemmas, problem-solving, communications, relationships, and ourselves as individuals" (Anderson & Burney, 1996, p. 4). Anderson highlighted the role of curiosity in a conversational partnership:

> Dialogue requires an openness to the other and their differences as well as openness to being questioned, critiqued, and not agreed with. What is important is to try to understand from the other's sense-making or logic map, not from yours.
>
> *(2016, p. 13)*

Thus a C-D practitioner should be immensely curious about the client's life, and act from a learning position.

The conversational partnership is favored and may be nurtured by: (1) a warm demeanor, (2) an attitude of interest, (3) a learning position, and (4) a yearning to understand (Anderson, 2007e, p. 45). This is *withness* in action. A therapist is genuinely interested in the client's worldview and follows what the client wants to discuss and how they want to share it. Therapists do not mandate the format a client must use to share information, but, inevitably, the conversation itself takes on a natural flow toward a certain direction.

Drawing from the vocabulary of modernist family therapists like Salvador Minuchin, just by partaking in the conversation, the therapist is "manipulative" in the sense that they maneuver the conversation. But in C-DP, the therapist is not manipulative in the sense that therapists aim for certain outcomes through tactics or directives. In other words, a therapist cannot *not* be an influence, but they can choose to avoid skillful deception, tactics, techniques, or directives that limit the ways the client can *be* or share information intuitively.

A C-D therapist sets any preconceived agenda aside, listens assiduously, converses reflexively through verbal and non-verbal language, asks clarifying questions, allows room for natural silences, and checks in with their client throughout the session (Anderson, 2007f). In practice, being a conversational partner means maintaining an open stance that lends to natural dialogue. Again, we often do this outside of the therapy room when the conversation "flows." Ideally, the conversation generates new meanings and understandings for the partners. Hence, the dialogue is described as *generative* (for its creation of new meanings) and *transformative* (for the impact it has on participants). This means that it is not the therapist who changes the client or client's actions. The therapist is also changed during these transformative dialogues; it works both ways, with each person walking away from the conversation with a new understanding, sometimes different values, and a changed reality (e.g., Anderson, 2001).

Maintain personal and professional congruency

Anderson and Goolishian's philosophical approach is unique in many ways. It "requires a mindset shift that gives us the freedom to uniquely interact and respond with each other in ways congruent with the person and the occasion" (Anderson, 2023a, p. 25). As Anderson discussed with her interviewer (Malinen), there is a consistency in who the therapist is inside and outside of the therapy room. Unlike the common modernist family therapist predicament, you do not measure how much of your personality to bring into your role as the therapist because you are bringing your*self* into the room, 100% of you, because you *are* the "model"—if you will—when you embody these social constructionist beliefs and practices. This is a philosophical way of life, and when you embrace it, you can see that any division between a *personal you* and a *professional you* is an illusion. C-DP is a "philosophy of life that forms and informs both a professional and personal way of being in the world: the two cannot be separated" (Anderson, 2007e, p. 43).

> The values I carry with me, the way I handle myself, my style, and so on, there's a congruency in that. Sometimes people have the idea when you go into the therapy room, you have to totally change: You have a white coat and a list of questions, you behave a certain way called "professional."
>
> *(Anderson, 2012b, p. 81)*

Therapists and their directors, supervisors, colleagues, and peers will each have varied, multifaceted ideas about what therapy is and what a therapy session should look like. Having fought to be taken seriously as "more than just talking," it is unsurprising that the mental health community encourages professionalism. But what is professionalism? What makes one therapist professional while another is not? There is intersectionality here. Morality, ethics, and legality are all separate domains. Add in professionalism, and we have a fourth. As you ask yourself, "What are my expectations for myself as a therapist?" and, "What should I do?" consider what motivates your answer. Remember that postmodernism is skeptical of metanarratives, so it is insufficient to say, "I am supposed to do 'x,' 'y,' or 'z.'" According to whom? To whose idea of professionalism are you adhering? Anderson's ideal professional is one who is congruent across different spheres of their life, not one who is one way with clients and a totally different way outside of the therapy room. Yes, we all have our different hats. But we each know from experience when we are slightly different because of our contextual environment and when we are pretending, posturing, or performing based on what we think is expected of us.

Use local language

Local language is "the unique wisdom created and used within a community of persons" (Anderson, 2014, p. 65). Because "therapists often lose touch with the client's locally developed meanings and can constrain the client's narrative" (Anderson & Goolishian, 1988, p. 33), a C-D practitioner makes sure to attend to the client's personal beliefs and knowledges rather than push a private agenda for the client (Anderson & Gehart, 2023).

C-D practitioners refrain from presuppositions about the client's story or the meaning behind their story, and the story is embraced in their "local language" (Malinen), meaning their natural, unpretentious language that fits with their culture and context. Rather than educating the client on professional terminology that the client should use, C-D practitioners push themselves to adopt the client's language and see how the clients are using words, consistently checking in that they understand the client's language. Local language is the relaxed, naturally flowing language the client would use. Contrast this to jargon-heavy conversations where the client almost becomes a pupil forced to memorize a psychological lexicon. We are quick to jump to jargon. In such cases where you are tempted, ask yourself who the jargon is for. Do clients really need to memorize a definition of "symmetrical escalation," "differentiation," or "double-bind" for example?

You can see how the therapist privileging the client's worldview fits with a reasoning that the therapist might learn the client's language instead of teaching the client mental health terms. The client is not taking the licensure exam, and there is often no need to introduce therapeutic jargon into the conversation when regular words will do. C-DP is an alternative approach to traditional (i.e., modernist) therapy such as psychoeducation-focused or diagnostic-oriented sessions that rely on teaching the client.

Co-explore, co-develop, and collaborate

The theory of change in Anderson's model is that change happens in dialogue. However, given the previous connotations of the word "change" in modernist family therapy models and Anderson's desire to separate from the modernist lineage, Anderson preferred to use the word "transformation" instead (Hoff & Anderson). As we touched upon earlier, transformation happens in and through *dialogical conversations*, a mutually influencing conversation rather than a prescribed intervention. Dialogical conversations are a dance of *withness* and speaking and listening—unsurprisingly—collaboratively (Anderson, 2007c, p. 25). It requires a certain amount of intentionality, letting go of rigid opinions, and making space for multiple (even contradictory) voices, and it is frequently more difficult for therapists who have preconceived notions of what therapy "should" look like (Anderson, 2007a, 2012a, 2016; Gehart, 2023; Hoffman).

Anderson described dialogical conversations as "a generative process in which new meanings—different ways of understanding, making sense of, or punctuating one's lived experiences—emerge and are mutually constructed" (1997, p. 108). Transformation takes place in and through these dialogical conversations (where knowledge is communally constructed) (Hoff & Anderson). Since language constructs, as the language evolves, the story evolves, and thus reality evolves (Anderson, 2007e; Anderson & Goolishian, 1991). Previously held assumptions can be questioned. Each person is affected by the conversation. Remember, a therapist from a C-DP view is neither waiting for nor trying to get the client to agree with the therapist or see the therapist's perspective. To reiterate Anderson's key point, transformation happens in dialogical conversations, not *monological conversations.*

You may be familiar with the term monologue from theater where one person speaks for an uninterrupted block of time. Colloquially, a monologue is typically associated with someone who tends to dominate the conversation, often without allowing an opportunity for others' voices. The concept of *"dialogical vs monological"* speaking parallels *"withness vs aboutness"* speaking (Hoffman, p. 10). As Goolishian and Anderson said, "In monologue, no new meaning arises. One perspective reigns, and reality becomes closed" (Goolishian & Anderson, 1987, p. 532).

Traditional therapists tend to go into "advice mode" or "fix-it mode," which are forms of monologue. Likewise, a client who speaks continuously for 50 minutes while the therapist says nothing would also be engaging in a monologue. You can see how neither dynamic in a therapist-client relationship would be conducive to transformation.

Gergen added that monologue is self-isolating (Gergen et al., 1996). Anderson echoed his sentiment, adding that conversational partners can get into *dueling monologues,* which lead to *dueling realities* where neither party lets go of their position enough to be curious about the other's (Anderson, 2012b; Gergen, Hoffman, & Anderson). Anderson normalized different voices having different perspectives without them competing (e.g., 2012a).

You may think about dueling monologues as a debate and dialogical conversations as a philosophical position. In a debate, each person tries to convince the other of the correctness of their position. In a dialogical conversation, you philosophically explore ideas together to reach new conclusions. Listening attentively and nondefensively is critical. Anderson highlighted the openness of a dialogical conversation as "a mutual or shared inquiry in an interactive and fluid process in which therapist and client co-explore the familiar and co-develop the new" (Anderson, 2001, p. 349).

With the right balance of give-and-take, open listening, contemplative reflection, and genuine presence, monologues can become dialogues. *Withness* conversations become transformative dialogues. *Transformative dialogues* are conversations that generate new meanings out of the "back-and-forthness" (Anderson, 2007a) of the joint, relational exchange. New ideas emerge and participants are transformed by what transpires.

> A dialogical conversation is a two-way conversation, a back-and-forth, give-and-take, in-there-together process where people talk *with* rather than *to* each other. Inviting this kind of partnership requires that the client's story take center stage. It requires that the therapist constantly learn, listening to and trying to understand the client's story from the client's perspective. The therapist is listening to hear what the understanding is for the client, not for the therapist.
>
> *(Anderson, 2001, p. 348)*

For a dialogue to be transformative, it must be a spur-of-the-moment co-creation of new knowledges and realities for the therapist and client which leave lasting impressions on both such that they are different people before and after the conversation. The conversation itself opens space for new possibilities and new narratives, expanding stories and facilitating self-agency (Anderson & Burney, 1996).

Thinking of engaging in this type of dialogue as a technique is reductive (Anderson, 2016) and misses the mark. As Anderson (2023a) astutely noted, "People want step-by-step recipes for how to do dialogue, and many practitioners have been happy to deliver them" (p. 25). However, her stance requires both more and less of the therapist. It requires less pre-planned, prescribed, anticipated, or orchestrated interventions and agendas; meanwhile, it requires more presence and cultivation of "the art of *withness*" in navigating spontaneous therapeutic conversations (Anderson, 2007a).

Be "public"

> I started to use the term or the words *"being public."* It refers to the commitment and activity of not operating from hidden or private ideas, thoughts, questions, but rather being open and making them visible. Though I keep in mind that regardless of what I choose to show other persons, what they see or hear and how they interpret it will be uniquely theirs, not mine.
>
> *(Anderson, 2012b, p. 68)*

Because the aim is to have transformative dialogical conversations, a C-D therapist also avoids internal monologues. If a therapist is engaging in an internal thought or idea that continuously loops in their head, it takes them out of the present moment of being in a two-way dialogical conversation. The therapist cannot lead with genuine, authentic, "withness-type" curiosity if they are waiting for their turn to speak, thinking of what question to ask next, or doubting the truthfulness or integrity of the client.

> Therapists often learn to operate from invisible private inner thoughts—professionally, personally, theoretically, or experientially informed inner talk—understandings such as diagnoses, judgments, or hypotheses. These thoughts can influence how the therapist listens and hears and can guide the therapist's questions and responses. From a collaborative (i.e., C-DP) stance, therapists are open and make their invisible thoughts visible. The therapist may share any idea—for instance, an opinion, question, or suggestion—with the client. The intent of the sharing or being public with one's inner thoughts is to offer them as food for thought and dialogue.
>
> *(2012a, p. 281)*

Anderson's concept of being public is getting internal thoughts out so you both can talk about them transparently, much like Tom Andersen's practice (Anderson, 2012b; Anderson & Goolishian, 1991). It may be helpful to initially conceptualize *being public* as avoiding getting lost in a sea of internal thoughts like secret hypotheses, secret perceived solutions, or secret goals. The act/art of being public opens space for new possibilities in dialogue. Although not exactly the same, there is some overlap here with self-disclosure. If part of the internal monologue is self-disclosure-related and a therapist weighs the pros and cons and decides the information they might share could be useful food for thought without harm, they share it. How they share it is important. Rather than assume a modernist position of a "boundary violation," a C-D therapist sees merit to sharing authentically. Anything is on the table as long as it is *not* presented as a fact. The more useful presentation of the thought is, as I learned to say, "just an idea" or as Anderson liked to say, "food for thought." Although not the intention, I find being public reinforces to my clients that I am trustworthy and able to cherish the vulnerability they share.

Employ a non-expert, not-knowing stance

"Agnostic" is a term derived from the ancient Greek roots "-A" (without) + "GNOSIS" (knowledge; pronounced "know-sis"). In a religious sense, agnostic refers to someone who does not know if God exists or not and does not confirm nor deny the existence of a god or gods, a universal being, and so on. For a moment, consider this term outside of a religious context. C-DP encourages us to consider becoming "agnostic" practitioners, acting from a place where we do not know what a client should or should not do and cannot speak to the ways that it is best for them to live their life.

A key part of the C-D practitioner's role is to maintain a *non-expert stance*, which is a belief that the client is the expert on their own life, not the therapist. Any ideas or preconceived notions or identity conclusions like, "She's a boredom-making machine" (Malinen, 2004, p. 69), or labeling someone as "a difficult client," "a treatment failure," or "a revolving door case"—as Anderson's colleagues said about her clients (Hoff & Anderson)—are off the table. Those thoughts stem from a modernist stance where the therapist assumes they are the expert and can achieve a better or more inclusive view of the problem than the client—the "God's eye view," as Gergen called it. A non-expert stance means the therapist does not assume they have a privileged view of the problem, individual, couple, or family.

When Anderson and Goolishian introduced the "*not-knowing stance,*" they received uproarious feedback from modernist mental health professionals. But worry not; the not-knowing stance does not mean a therapist accrued student loan debt for nothing. Nor does Anderson's not-knowing stance mean we forget everything we have ever learned about therapy or that we leave our biases and values at the door (which social constructionists believe is impossible to do). Instead, it refers to "a way to think about knowing: about what I know or what I think I might know, and the intent with which I offer that knowledge as well as the intent with which I use it" (Anderson, 2012b, p. 67). It is a genuine stance, and unlike MRI's "one-down position," it is not a posture one displays but a belief one chooses to adopt.

Not-knowing is simply where the therapist does not know or "pre-know." Oftentimes, therapists are taught to come up with hypotheses, sometimes even before meeting clients, based on intake paperwork. The not-knowing stance is the antithesis of that. Anderson and Goolishian cautioned against "understanding or knowing too quickly [which] interferes with listening" (1991, p. 25). They explained:

> Premature assumptions and questions can limit the telling of the client's story and can limit access to the opportunity for new stories, new meanings, and new agency. Additionally, if the therapist's preconceived ideas and knowledge set the parameters of the client's story, then therapy is less than a collaborative process (p. 25).

The not-knowing stance blends seamlessly into the *non-expert stance*. The therapist is the expert on how to facilitate a dialogue but is not the expert on the client's life.

> Instead of being an expert on the client (including their problem, resources, preferred solutions, etc.), the therapist's competence or expertise is in establishing and fostering an environment and condition that naturally invites collaborative relationships and generative conversational processes.
>
> *(Anderson, 2007e, p. 46)*

When a practitioner truly believes: (1) the therapist does not see a clearer or more complete picture of the situation than the client, (2) the therapist does not have to come up with the answer for the client, (3) the therapist does not have to steer clients toward a certain course or outcome, (4) the client knows their own life better than the therapist, and (5) each client is unique in their circumstances rather than belonging to a type or category of client or problem; they are well on their way to acting from C-DP's non-expert, not-knowing stance. When you bring your full self into the room, it is impossible for a therapist to be "neutral" (Anderson, 1997), but quite possible to take on multiple, even contradictory, positions at the same time. The key in all of this is to allow yourself to be a listener instead of a judge.

> The client is the expert on their story and the contents of the story. The client is the expert on what's important and what's not important to talk about. When I think of the client as the expert, that makes me the learner. The client is my teacher, and I'm learning from them.
>
> *(Anderson, 2012b, p. 66)*

As you can see, this connects to a *non-hierarchical* stance as well. Privileging the client's worldview above your own, allowing yourself to be informed by your client's expertise, and being a host/guest turn the tables on modernist expectations. The therapist cannot "eliminate" hierarchy but chooses to lower the hierarchy even though a therapist is technically in a position of power in relation to the client. This way, the therapist and client are more egalitarian than in a traditional, modernist therapist-client relationship; however, the therapist is aware of the inherent power dynamic. This is the answer, or at least my answer, to Anderson's question about what makes a dinner table conversation between friends different than a therapeutic conversation. The power dynamic between friends is not the same as between clients. However, the authentic conversational connection can be, more or less, the same. This means that when your modernist supervisor criticizes you for allowing your client to go on a tangent or accuses your clients of being evasive, you can politely correct their well-intentioned misunderstanding of your epistemology. If you are operating from C-DP's non-expert, non-hierarchical, not-knowing stance, "withness wandering" is part of the process. You trust that the important information will come out and be returned to organically. You trust the process. Your expertise translates as a facilitator of the dialogical process rather than an expert on what the client should do.

A lack of goals

This emphasis on the dialogical process means that one must change their conceptualization of goals: what they are and their purpose in therapy. There are no goals in this type of therapy—at least not in the traditional, modernist sense (Hoff & Anderson, 2016). Most traditional therapists think of problems as concrete and solutions as concrete. We even have something called SMART goals in the psychotherapy community, which stand for "Specific, Measurable, Achievable, Realistic, and Timely" goals. C-D therapists instead have malleable agendas; they have a direction they head toward but not a specific path and certainly no concrete boxes that need to be ticked off. The "success" of a therapeutic conversation is in each person's genuine, meticulous listening, openness, and creating space for new possibilities and shifts (Anderson & Goolishian, 1991).

In much the same way the "goal" of a conversation with a friend or colleague can change as the conversation naturally progresses, the goal of therapy can change. Here, we throw out the modernist assumption that we need to fix clients' problems by suggesting the perfect solution, introducing a paradoxical task to disrupt patterns, and so on. Anderson talked about problems being simply "dis-solved" in conversation. In her seminal work, she said,

> *Solution* has the connotation of fixing. I believe that a therapist or therapy neither *solves* problems nor fixes anything. In my experience, that does not happen; rather, problem exploration in the therapy process leads to problem dissolution, not problem solution. Problems are not solved but dissolved ("dis-solved") in language. In my view, the process through which you talk about something, not its content (for instance, problems or solutions), is the significant factor.
>
> *(1997, p. 91)*

The dissolution of the problem would, by modernist standards, be the goal. However, to dis-solve the problem might involve talking differently about the problem, and it might involve talking about things outside the problem. Certainly, new thoughts might stem from the conversation, but there are no criteria that those thoughts need to fulfill. What C-DP therapists find most useful is humility, non-judgment, and compassion in a moment-by-moment awareness of and participation in a transformative, dialogical conversation (see Gehart, 2023, pp. 66–70).

SUMMARY

Taking a tentative stance toward Truth, this approach values the community construction of knowledge and sees truths as communally created in language. Anderson and Goolishian's approach holds space for the client and does not make presumptuous claims to pre-knowing or pre-understanding. It encourages every member involved to be authentic, and therapists allow themselves to be informed by the clients rather than the other way around. The non-expert, not-knowing stance is neither an act nor a technique. Because everyone has a seat at the table, the therapeutic experience is empowering for all those partaking in such special conversations, and each person is transformed by being a genuine part of it. Their presence transforms the dialogical conversation; meanwhile, they are transformed by taking part in the dialogical conversation. Transformative dialogue creates new knowledges, new meanings, and new realities for clients. When the therapist is *with* the client, the therapist is open to being transformed by the conversation too, which allows both parties to be mutually changed by the dialogue.

Anderson does not think that people are broken; therefore, there is no "fixing" them. Rather than a modernist concept of behavioral goals and milestones to achieve, Anderson is more interested in the family's shifting agenda. It may behoove therapists to think of it this way: one can have a tentative agenda and be willing to adjust in accordance with where the conversation naturally goes. In this way, the collaborative therapist adopts a position of uncertainty and spontaneity (Malinen).

C-DP is arguably the "most postmodern" and "least manipulative" of the family therapy models, believing in infinite realities, having flexible agendas instead of concrete goals and being open to changing course without prior notice. This not-model (remember, it is a *philosophy*) is one where intent matters. A C-D therapist is authentically themselves in their being and in their conversations. There is no duplicity in this model, as the thoughts the therapist shares with the client are authentic. There are no paradoxical interventions where the therapist says one thing but hopes the client will do another.

I see C-DP as a straightforward model. Rather than having your takeaway be that you need to "do," think of it ontologically first: you need to "be." And in being a certain way (specifically a social constructionist who adopts a not-knowing stance), things will naturally happen. Then you can work on refining your ability to facilitate transformative dialogue. The process of "dialoguing" is an art, not a science.

REFLECTIVE QUESTIONS

1. Why might Anderson describe what she does as being polite?
2. How does one be a polite "host-guest" with a client?
3. Can you think of times when you were practicing "withness" but perhaps did not know it?
4. What is the expected outcome from a C-DP dialogue?
5. How might C-DP conflict with the modernist psychotherapeutic systems in which most of us work?

Keywords

Collaborative Language Systems (CLS)
Collaborative-Dialogic Practice (C-DP)
Language Systems Theory
Social Constructionism
Hermeneutics
"Withness"
"Both/And"
Mutual Puzzling
Host-Guest
Conversational Partner
Local Language
Dialogical Conversations
Transformative Dialogues
Being Public
Non-Expert Stance
Not-Knowing Stance

Collaborative Dialogic Practice Post-Test (Inspired by Anderson, 1997)

1. What is the therapist's position in relation to the clients?
   a. A therapist adopts a non-hierarchical position.

2. How does the therapist's academic learning and site training come into play?
   a. The therapist has certain knowledge and expertise; it does not cancel out or overshadow the clients' expertise on their own lives.
3. Does a therapist listen for facts, patterns, or stories (or something else)?
   a. A therapist asks the clients what they think is important for the therapist to hear.
4. Is the therapist a subject-matter expert?
   a. The therapist is an expert at transformative dialogue, not a content-subject-matter expert. Therapists can bring in their own ideas, but they are offered as "food for thought," not facts.
5. To what extent should a therapist know what the client should do?
   a. A therapist adopts a not-knowing stance and waits to be informed by their clients. Polite suggestions may be tentatively offered if the client says they want to hear their therapist's ideas. The therapist introduces these to see if they resonate with the client and is not attached to their suggestions; they are not affected negatively in any way (e.g., disappointed, discouraged, annoyed, or defensive) if the client does not follow through with the suggestion.
6. How important is it to identify causality? How important is it to discuss causality with your clients?
   a. Not at all. The therapist does not think in terms of causality; they listen for the ways their clients weave their stories together. This opens space for creativity and new possibilities that may not have been considered.
7. What should a therapist be certain about?
   a. A therapist would embrace uncertainty, which is often more difficult than acting from a place of certainty. There is a not-knowing, wait-to-be-informed stance.
8. What information, thoughts, and opinions should be shared with clients? What should not be shared?
   a. The therapist holds their own beliefs, opinions, and values. Those are put on the backburner, so to speak, as the therapist engages in transformative dialogue and those enter at the therapist's discretion as "being public."
9. How important is it that the therapist has an extensive toolkit with techniques and strategies?
   a. A therapist does not employ techniques or strategies. Questions and comments are authentically curious and are not meant to lead the client to certain conclusions. The whole therapeutic process of engaging in a transformative dialogue is the closest thing, yet this is a genuine philosophical stance, not a method or procedure.
10. How does a therapist produce or induce change?
    a. The therapist does not induce change in the client. Both therapist and client are transformed by a dialogical conversation but, as Harry Goolishian said, "the only person a therapist can change is themself" (Anderson, 1997, p. 125).
11. What is the "self"?
    a. Selves are relational and in language, not inside an individual.
12. What is important for a therapist to investigate?
    a. Therapists are neither interrogators nor detectives. They engage in mutual inquiry as they co-create knowledge with clients in collaborative-dialogical conversation.

HARLENE ANDERSON AND HARRY GOOLISHIAN: PRIMARY SOURCES

Anderson, H. (1984). *The new epistemology in family therapy: Implications for training family therapists.* The Union for Experimenting Colleges and Universities.

Anderson, H. (1996). Reflection on client-professional collaboration. *Families, Systems, & Health, 14*(2), 193–206.

Anderson, H. (1997). *Conversation, language, and possibilities: A postmodern approach to therapy.* Basic Books.

Anderson, H. (2001). Postmodern collaborative and person-centered therapies: What would Carl Rogers say? *Journal of Family Therapy, 23,* 339–360.

Anderson, H. (2007a). Creating a space for a generative community. In H. Anderson & P. Jensen (Eds.), *Innovations in the reflecting process* (pp. 33–45, dig. ed.). Routledge.

Anderson, H. (2007b). Dialogue: People creating meaning with each other and finding ways to go on. In H. Anderson & D. Gehart (Eds.), *Collaborative therapy: Relationships and conversations that make a difference* (pp. 33–42, dig. ed.). Routledge.

Anderson, H. (2007c). Historical influences. In H. Anderson & D. Gehart (Eds.), *Collaborative therapy: Relationships and conversations that make a difference* (pp. 21–32, dig. ed.). Routledge.

Anderson, H. (2007d). Postmodern umbrella: Language and knowledge as relational and generative and inherently transforming. In H. Anderson & D. Gehart (Eds.), *Collaborative therapy: Relationships and conversations that make a difference* (pp. 7–20, dig. ed.). Routledge.

Anderson, H. (2007e). The heart and spirit of collaborative therapy: The philosophical stance—"A way of being" in relationship and conversation. In H. Anderson & D. Gehart (Eds.), *Collaborative therapy: Relationships and conversations that make a difference* (pp. 43–59, dig. ed.). Routledge.

Anderson, H. (2007f). The therapist and the postmodern therapy system: A way of being *with* others. *6th Congress of the European Family Therapy Association and 32nd Association for Family Therapy and Systemic Practice UK Conference.* Glasgow, Scotland. October 5, 2007. https://europeanfamilytherapy.eu/wp-content/uploads/anderson.pdf

Anderson, H. (2012a). Collaborative relationships and dialogic conversations: Ideas for a relationally responsive practice. *Family Process, 51,* 8–24.

Anderson, H. (2012b). Possibilities of the collaborative approach. In T. Malinen, S. J. Cooper, & F. N. Cooper (Eds.), *Masters of narrative and collaborative therapies: The voices of Andersen, Anderson, and White* (pp. 61–120, dig. ed.). Routledge.

Anderson, H. (2014). Collaborative-dialogue based research as everyday practice questioning our myths. In G. Simon & A. Chard (Eds.), *Systemic inquiry: Innovations in reflexive practice research* (pp. 60–73). Everything is Connected Press.

Anderson, H. (2016). Listening, hearing and speaking: Brief thoughts on the relationship to dialogue. *Psychological Opinions, 7,* 10–14.

Anderson, H. (2023a). Conceptual framework: Emerging orienting sensitivities for relationships and conversations that invite transformation and possibility. In H. Anderson & D. R. Gehart (Eds.), *Collaborative-dialogic practice: Relationships and conversations that make a difference across contexts and cultures* (pp. 19–33, dig. ed.). Routledge.

Anderson, H. (2023b). Expressions of the philosophical stance: Creating a relational and dialogic space and process for generativity. In H. Anderson & D. R. Gehart (Eds.), *Collaborative-dialogic practice: Relationships and conversations that make a difference across contexts and cultures* (pp. 34–49, dig. ed.). Routledge.

Anderson, H., & Burney, J. P. (1996). Collaborative inquiry: A postmodern approach to organizational consultation. *Human Systems: The Journal of Systemic Consultation and Management, 7*(2-3), 171–188.

Anderson, H., & Gehart, D. R. (Eds.). (2023). *Collaborative-dialogic practice: Relationships and conversations that make a difference across contexts and cultures* (dig. ed.). Routledge.

Anderson, H., & Gehart, D. (Eds.). (2007). *Collaborative therapy: Relationships and conversations that make a difference* (dig. ed.). Routledge.

Anderson, H., & Goolishian, H. (1988). Human systems as linguistic systems: Evolving ideas about the implications for theory and practice. *Family Process, 27,* 371–393.

Anderson, H., & Goolishian, H. (1991). Thinking about multi-agency work with substance abusers and their families: A language systems approach. *Journal of Systemic Therapies, 10*(1), 20–35.

Anderson, H., & Goolishian, H. (1992). The client is the expert: A not-knowing approach to therapy. In S. McNamee & K. J. Gergen (Eds.), *Constructing therapy: Social construction and the therapeutic process* (pp. 25–36). Sage.

Anderson, H., Goolishian, H. A., & Windermand, L. (1986). Problem determined systems: Towards transformation in family therapy. *Journal of Strategic and Systemic Therapies, 5*(4), 1–13.

Anderson, H., & Jenson, P. (2007). Preface. In H. Anderson & P. Jensen (Eds.), *Innovations in the reflecting process* (pp. xix–xxi, dig. ed.). Routledge.

Gergen, K. J., Hoffman, L., & Anderson, H. (1996). Is diagnosis a disaster: A constructionist trialogue. In F. Kaslow (Ed.), *Relational diagnosis* [draft]. Wiley.

Goolishian, H., & Anderson, H. (1987). Language systems and therapy: An evolving idea. *Psychotherapy, 24*(3), 529–538.

Hoff, C., & Anderson, H. (2016, March 20). Collaborative-Dialogic practice and the postmodern perspective [Audio podcast episode]. In *The Radical Therapist.* Podbean. https://chrishoffmft.podbean.com/e/the-radical-therapist-017---collaborative-dialogic-practice-and-the-postmodern-perspective-w-harlene-anderson-phd/

Renowned Sources

Andersen, T. (2007). Human participating: Human "being" is the next step to human "becoming" in the next step. In In H. Anderson & D. Gehart (Eds.), *Collaborative therapy* (pp. 81–93, dig. ed.). Routledge.

Andersen, T. (2012). Words—Universes traveling by. In T. Malinen, S. J. Cooper, & F. N. Cooper (Eds.), *Masters of narrative and collaborative therapies: The voices of Andersen, Anderson, and White* (pp. 61–120, dig. ed.). Routledge.

Gehart, D. R. (2023). Curiosity as mindfulness practice: Following the moment-to-moment unfolding of meaning construction. In H. Anderson & D. R. Gehart (Eds.), *Collaborative-dialogic practice: Relationships and conversations that make a difference across contexts and cultures* (pp. 66–79, dig. ed.). Routledge.

Gehart, D., Tarragona, M., & Bava, S. (2007). A collaborative approach to research and inquiry. In H. Anderson & D. Gehart (Eds.), *Collaborative therapy: Relationships and conversations that make a difference* (pp. 367–389, dig. ed.). Routledge.

Haley, J. (2010). *Uncommon therapy: The psychiatric techniques of Milton Erickson.* W. W. Norton.

Hoffman, L. (2007). Practicing "withness": A human art. In H. Anderson & P. Jensen (Eds.), *Innovations in the reflecting process* (pp. 3–15, dig. ed.). Routledge.

Malinen, T. (2004). The wisdom of not-knowing: A conversation with Harlene Anderson. *Journal of Systemic Therapies, 23*(2), 68–77.

Shotter, J. (2007). Not to forget Tom Andersen's way of being Tom Andersen: The importance of what 'just happens' to us. *Human Systems: The Journal of Systemic Consultation & Management, 18,* 15–28.

Additional References

Camus, A. (1986). *L'Hôte.* Hueber.

Sidis, A. E., Moore, A. R., Pickard, J., & Deane, F. P. (2022). "Always opening and never closing": How dialogical therapists understand and create reflective conversations in network. *Frontiers Psychology, 13,* 992785.

Kenneth (Ken) Gergen

....

Remember, as you read through these chapters, you can always return to the Introduction to refresh your memory on the terms you learned such as epistemology, ontology, positivism, Cartesian dualism, and social constructionism.

QUESTIONS TO THINK ABOUT

1. What are the seminal texts associated with Ken Gergen?
2. How does Gergen's philosophy challenge positivism and Cartesian dualism?
3. What makes a conversation generative and/or transformative?
4. What is the relationship between language and reality?

Chapter 1 introduced collaborative-dialogic practice (C-DP). Chapter 2 explores the American social psychologist and philosopher Ken Gergen's epistemology and important philosophical ideas which inspired not only Harlene Anderson and Harry Goolishian, but also other postmodern family therapists. Ken Gergen's biggest gift to family therapy and qualitative research is *social constructionism*.

> Social constructionist inquiry is principally concerned with explicating the processes by which people come to describe, explain, or otherwise account for the world (including themselves) in which they live. It attempts to articulate the common forms understanding as they now exist, as they have existed in prior historical periods, and as they might exist should creative attention be so directed.
>
> *(Gergen, 1985, p. 266)*

DOI: 10.4324/9781003439349-4

Because social constructionism is itself a socially constructed category, there can be no succinct definition that encapsulates social constructionism in any definite way; however, people generally agree that social constructionism is an epistemological paradigm that varies across cultures and time (Gergen, 2023). More specifically, social constructionism maintains that people cannot access an objective, singular reality; consequently, our knowledge cannot be derived from an ultimate source nor transferred to another. Subsequently, knowledge is constructed relationally in communities rather than derived from an ultimate Truth or Reality.

With the dominant culture in the United States being hyper-focused on things being valid or worth attention only if they can be proved through objective, specific, scientific processes, Gergen's ideas are often unsettling, contentious, or profane to modernists and a breath of fresh air to postmodernists. Social constructionist ideas like (1) *we do not have direct access to reality*, (2) *there are multiple realities*, and (3) *there is no objective knowledge* are still considered scandalous to many if not most.

As you can clearly see from my writing style, a social constructionist stance resonates with me, not a modernist lens. Yet Gergen's social constructionism is just one lens. Since our lenses are all constructs, I can certainly not claim Gergen's is best. However, I can say that a social constructionist stance resonates with me in a way modernism never did. Before I had the language to describe it, I would say, "Most people see the world as black and white, whereas I see gray." Social constructionism gave me the language to describe how I already saw the world. Clearly, Gergen's views are useful for me, personally and professionally. Perhaps social constructionism will resonate with you as it does me. It is a very culturally aware and inclusive philosophy. This is because of how social constructionism views language, views social processes, views communities, and views "the self." Language is viewed as constructing our reality, so conversations have the ability to change our worldviews. Pushing the envelope too far for some: we are different people before versus after a transformative dialogue. Social processes are viewed as a complex series of actions. Rather than be structure-focused, these processes are conceptualized as very human, so individuals are in a complex web of interconnection.

Like in the previous chapter, I encourage you to read this with an open mind and see what internal dialogues happen as you step into social constructionist ideas. An understanding of social constructionism will allow you to practice C-DP, narrative therapy, or solution focused brief therapy (SFBT). Beyond this, an understanding of social constructionism can allow for new possibilities in your own life—new ways of living and practicing therapy.

WHO IS KEN GERGEN?

Kenneth J. Gergen (pronounced with two hard "G's": "GRR-GNN") is an eminent, postmodern social psychologist and social constructionist whose philosophy spans across disciplines including research, psychology, and family therapy. His interest is not in the physical world that he believes we cannot directly access but in the relational world from which he believes we cannot escape (Gergen, 2023). His works emphasize language, communication, and social interaction.

Ken Gergen was married to Mary Gergen, an American feminist social psychologist, until she passed away in 2020. They collaborated over the years, writing about constructionism, social constructionism, and feminist ideas. Mary Gergen built a reputation as an activist and published on some of her interests, including aging, women and gender studies, and LGBTQ+ issues (Gergen, 2023; Gergen & Gergen, 2002). Like the founder of narrative therapy Michael White, Ken and Mary Gergen were extremely interested in relational and communal influences on people's ways of living—their knowledges, beliefs, and values.

> It is within communal interchange that we come to develop both ontologies and ethics. We come to share languages in which certain distinctions are made and not others and in which value comes to be placed on these distinctions and the actions in which they are embedded. Thus we find enormous cultural differences in world constructions and their associated values, and also within these cultures striking differences among sub-cultures.... As the same language is circulated among people, actions are coordinated around this language, trust is developed, dissenting voices are eliminated, others are identified as "outside" the circle, and those outside are increasingly disparaged.
>
> *(Gergen, 2003, p. 108)*

Recall from the Introduction how if you are a social constructionist, you necessarily believe in multiple realities and multiple truths. Now, not every person in a community or sub-community shares the same values, however, there will be a majority where most people in a given group come to an agreement on what people "should" do; this reveals what communities consider "good," "bad," "right," and "wrong." When this happens, outliers are "othered," to use a term from social theory, anthropology, and feminism. This means that people see individuals belonging to an "othered" group as fundamentally different and often inferior.

Building upon this understanding, the Gergen's each critiqued "The Realist Assumption" (Gergen, 1998, p. 2) and the inherent shortcomings of two systems of belief in traditional (i.e., modernist) thought: Cartesian dualism and positivism. You can revisit the Introduction if you need to refresh your memory on these terms. In brief, Descartes' quote, "I think, therefore I am" perpetuates an individualistic worldview where certainty (about existence) is derived by thinking. Descartes' focus is on the mind (thinking) prior to and separated from the body (being). Hence, the "brain-body divide" holds the mind on a different plane than the body.

Positivism, meanwhile, is criticized by postmodernists for its over-reliance on measurement and methods, frequently the scientific method, to establish "Truth." It reifies the idea that knowledge can only be acquired through empirical observation and testing, which marginalizes other means of knowing. By assuming one can (1) directly access reality and (2) access reality through testing hypotheses, we self-reinforce the idea of validity only belonging to the testable, observable, and quantifiable.

Taking issue with this, Ken Gergen (1985) said that social constructionism begins with "radical doubt" (p. 267) of our taken-for-granted assumptions, including those about "Science's" relationship with reality. Gergen (1985) explained that "what we take to be experience of the world does not itself dictate the terms by which the world is understood" (p. 266). Essentially, our understanding of the world is shaped by contextual factors such as culture, sub-culture, and history. Our experience of something, such as "time," we take to be objective; however, upon further review, time is a social construct, and individual experience of time depends on many factors. If you are having trouble thinking of time as relational and intersubjective rather than objective, ask yourself, "What time zone do I live in?"; "Is it daylight savings time?"; "Is time the same in memories and dreams?"; and so on.

Generally, postmodernists see these modernist approaches as contextualized without acknowledging their modernist cultural context and assumptions. This means that positivism and Cartesian dualism perpetuate understandings of Truth, not truths. Postmodernists, by definition, believe in truths (plural) rather than one Truth.

Postmodern philosopher Gergen offered a shift with his statement: "I am linked, therefore I am," which highlights seeing the world relationally instead of individualistically. This shift emphasizes a social constructionist view that people are interconnected. From this view, people engage in dynamic social processes that lead to the construction of meanings and identities. It discards the modernist notion of a "core self" (see Anderson, 2011). It points out the obvious: that we are different with different people across different realms. According to Gergen's philosophy, there is no static self. Furthermore, Gergen would say we are constantly defining and redefining ourselves in our interactions.

WHAT DID GERGEN WRITE?

Gergen, "one of the top 50 most influential living psychologists," has written over 300 books, magazines, and journal articles (The Taos Institute, 2023, para. 4). Two of his famous books are *An Invitation to Social Construction* (2023)—the first edition published in 1999—and *Relational Being: Beyond Self and Community* (2009a). These two books outlined social constructionist ideas as well as how one can imagine the individual within such a worldview.

Ken Gergen and Harlene Anderson have been engaged in a professional relationship since the early 1990s, after Anderson had first encountered his written words in 1985 (Anderson, 2011). In 1993, Harlene Anderson, David Cooperrider, Mary Gergen, Kenneth Gergen, Sheila McNamee, Suresh Srivastva, and Diana Whitney founded The Taos Institute in Taos, New Mexico. The Taos Institute created a space for theoretical and practical exploration of social constructionist ideas.

Both a part of the Silent Generation, Gergen and Anderson's dynamic is unique compared to the other philosophers and founders listed in this book. For example, White was part of the Baby Boomers, but his major philosophical influence (i.e., Foucault) belonged to the Greatest Generation. The founders of SFBT were part of the Silent Generation; however, a major philosophical influence on its postmodern development came from Ludwig Wittgenstein, a philosopher from the Lost Generation. As both Gergen and Anderson are living legends, it is clear their ideas mutually influenced and continue to influence each other.

TABLE 2.1 Through the generations

Generation	Date Ranges	Significant Person	Birth and Death Years
Unnamed Generation (I)	1820–1840	**Wilhelm Wundt** German Experimental Psychologist	b. 1832 d. 1920
Unnamed Generation (II)	1840–1960	**Sigmund Freud** Founder of Psychoanalysis	b. 1856 d. 1939
Unnamed Generation (III)	1860–1880	**Carl Jung** Psychoanalyst	b. 1875 d. 1961
Lost Generation	1880–1900	**Wittgenstein** Philosopher	b. 1889 d. 1951
Greatest Generation	1900–1925	**Harry Goolishian** Co-Founder of Collaborative-Dialogic Practice	b. 1924 d. 1991
		Michel Foucault Philosopher	b. 1926 d. 1984
Silent Generation	1925–1945	**Insoo Kim Berg** Co-Founder of Solution Focused Brief Therapy/ Steve's Partner	b. 1934 d. 2007
		Ken Gergen Philosopher/ Mary's Partner	b. 1934 -living
		Mary Gergen Social Psychologist/ Ken's Partner	b. 1938 d. 2020
		Steve de Shazer Co-Founder of Solution Focused Brief Therapy/ Insoo's Partner	b. 1940 d. 2005
		Harlene Anderson Co-Founder of Collaborative-Dialogic Practice	b. 1942 -living
		David Epston Co-Founder of Narrative Therapy	b. 1944 -living
Baby Boomers	1946–1964	**Michael White** Co-Founder of Narrative Therapy	b. 1948 d. 2008
Generation X	1965–1980		
Millennials (Gen Y)	1981–1996	(Your humble author)	
Generation Z	1997–2012		
Generation Alpha	2010–2025		

Note. There are no universally agreed upon date ranges for a given generation. The concept of a generation is a social construct. However, this table is based on the information provided by David Haas. (See references).

WHAT ARE GERGEN'S SOCIAL CONSTRUCTIONIST CONCEPTS?

> For present purposes we may see social constructionism as a range of dialogues centered on the social genesis of what we take to be knowledge, reason, and virtue, on the one side, and on the other the enormous range of social practices born and/or sustained by these discourses.
>
> *(Gergen, 2014, p. 131)*

Language as constructive

A modernist understanding of language is that language is a communication tool. You are likely familiar with this understanding if you were raised in a Western culture where language is largely considered representational. From this lens, language is understood to convey meanings. I think of this understanding like meanings being transported on a miniature model train track from Person A to Person B. Another frequently used simile is that language is like a mirror that reflects our thoughts, feelings, and ideas.

In contrast, a postmodernist, social constructionist understanding challenges the view that our language is representational or reflective like a mirror. "Social constructionism views discourse about the world not as a reflection or map of the world but as an artifact of communal interchange" (Gergen, 1985, p. 266). Social constructionists certainly would not agree that meaning can ever be conveyed or transported to another. From a social constructionist view, we are not passive recipients of language who wait for the train to arrive. We are more aptly seen as active participants in the creation of meaning who can never be outside of interpretation and the interpretation of interpretations. Therefore, constructs exist because language shapes and reshapes our realities, our relationships, our identities, and so on.

Social process

Social constructionism sees life as an inherently *social process* that cannot be extracted from the individual's culture, norms, and societal practices. Social constructionists argue that research, for example, is always influenced by the framework in which it is conducted. Research can never be objective or neutral, and researchers can never be outside observers. Culture—and the researcher's place in it—will always be a factor.

> For example, the scientist may use the most rigorous methods of testing intelligence and amass tomes of data that indicate racial differences in intelligence. However, to presume that there is something called "human intelligence," that people differ in their possession of this capacity, that there is something called "race," that race can be clearly determined, and that a series of question-and-answer games can reveal one's intelligence or race, is all specific to a given tradition or paradigm. Such concepts and measures are not required by "the way the world is." Most importantly, merely entering the paradigm and moving within the tradition is deeply injurious to those people classified as inferior by its standards. Or, to put it another way, the longstanding distinction between facts and

values—objective reflections of the world, and subjective desires or feelings of "ought"—cannot be sustained. Rather, values are intrinsic to facts.

(Gergen & Gergen, 2012, p. 68)

Life is too complicated, too interwoven to be able to be isolated and dissected, cut up into entities that supposedly result in getting "closer" to or even "arriving" at Truth. According to Gergen's philosophy of social constructionism: Truth itself is socially constructed.

Co-creation in communities

Gergen believes individuals are inextricably participating in the *co-action* or *co-creation* of knowledge in and through language. Social constructionist theory views language as fundamental to human understanding and meaning-making. Gergen influenced how one sees knowledge and reality as constructed through language rather than a reality to which we have pure access. Consider: (1) *What is language?*, (2) *What should we be aware of when we use language?*, and (3) *What is the impact of our language?*

Recalling our elephant allegory, Gergen claimed we do not have any unfiltered access to a pure reality. Gergen highlighted our predicament of always being in language: "When we search for the meaning of a word, we are thrust into an endless search through the dictionary. There is no exit to *the real*" (2023, p. 30). Gergen correspondingly referred to an idiosyncrasy in language called a tautology.

Tautology

Tautologies are a circular form of redundancy in language. There is a famous satiric play by Molière (pronounced "moh-lee-AIR") called *The Imaginary Invalid* (i.e., *Le Malade Imaginaire*). In this play, Molière wrote a comical exchange certain characters have about the "dormitive principle" of opium.

First Doctor

Very scholarly doctors,
Very famed assistants,
Very scholarly bachelor,
Whom I value and honor,
I ask you the reason and cause of why,
Why opium makes one sleep.

Bachelor

To me the scholarly doctor
Has asked the reason and cause of why,
Why opium makes one sleep.
To that I answer,
Because it contains in itself
Soporific properties
Whose nature it is to make one feel sleepy.

Chorus

Well, well, well answered.
Dignified and worthy to enter
Into our scholarly group.
Well answered.

So opium is soporific because it has soporific properties. In other words, it makes you sleepy because it has sleepy-making properties. This is a tautology. Gergen wrote, "Now ask yourself, what is reason outside this circle of mutual definition?" (2023, p. 31).

It is worth noting that Molière wrote the above exchange in a fake mixture of French and Latin. It is a common joke in Molière's satirical plays to have unintelligent people say simple things in a complicated way when they want to pretend to be clever. This excerpt makes fun of the pretentious professionals who prop their statements upon medical jargon, often Latin-based.

Generative discourses

Ken and Mary Gergen said that social constructionism "invites a *radical rationalism*" (Gergen & Gergen, 2012, p. 65). These two social psychologists shifted the focal point away from a modernist idea of *internal* toward a postmodern idea of *between*. They explained their postmodern alternative:

> In our view, an alternative view of human communication can indeed be drawn from the constructionist dialogues, not only as they are taking place within therapeutic circles, but as they have developed in the neighboring domains of ethnomethodology, the history of science, the sociology of knowledge, and literary theory. In each of these cases, there is a strong tendency to place the locus of meaning within the process of interaction itself. That is, the individual agent is de-emphasized as the source of meaning; attention moves from the *within* to the *between* (p. 72).

There is no meaning that "lies within" an individual. Meaning is co-constructed in communication. A high-five is dependent upon a recipient. If the recipient just entered on the other side of the room, it may be construed as a wave or greeting. If there is no other, the action is insignificant. Similarly, words do not *have* significance but *acquire* significance from co-action. Meaning lies within the interplay of co-action.

Conversations frequently involve shared language, eye-contact, silences, and laughter. If we are the speaker, we base our next move on the listener's response, and vice versa. Because of this, the Gergens believed conversations can best be described as a *generative* process. The participants collaborative in a process of seeking mutual understanding that involves interpretation and reinterpretation of a complex social interplay.

The exchange of ideas among individuals through dialogue will create (i.e., generate) subtle shifts that require new interpretations and understandings applied across domains. For example, in research the researchers build off one another's ideas, and their dialogue generates knowledge even before research participants are even introduced into the study. Their conversations change how they see the participants, the purpose of the study, the relationship of the study to truth and reality, and how they see one another. As the study evolves and conversations continue, interpretations necessarily change. It is important to realize that there are infinite interpretations, and as individuals come together in conversation, they collaborate in creating *an* interpretation—*a* reality.

Furthermore, the limits of any discourse enforce limits on reality. What we consider to be real is seen as a narrative in social constructionism. (Notably, "narrative" is not directly related to nor exclusive to narrative therapy). We cannot extend further than our reality, which is bounded by our intersubjective language.

In summary, social constructionism is oriented toward language, individuals' co-creation of meaning in communities, and the privileging of narratives over a so-called objective reality. Some key aspects of Gergen's social constructionist approach are to see it as:

1. A social practice;
2. A relational view of knowledge;
3. A path to multiple realities;
4. A narrative, discursive practice; and
5. Constrained and generated by language.

I end this section with Gergen's quote: "I cannot possess meaning alone" (Gergen & Gergen, 2012, p. 72).

BRIEF SUMMARIES AND ANALYSES OF GERGEN'S FAMOUS BOOKS

Relational being: beyond self and community (2009a)

Gergen argued against cause-and-effect accounts of behavior, which can be seen as crude and reductive. Cause and effect, a linear view, ignores the complexity of the relationship. He brought up the example of a game of billiards. The impact of the billiard stick is the cause, and the movement of the ball is the effect, yet, cause and effect are intricately intertwined and mutually shape each other, so "How can we identify a cause in itself, separated from an effect?" (p. 54). In a way, the effect determines (the meaning of and thus the reality of) the cause.

Actions within the context of human relationships and activities complicate things further. Consider his example of the socio-cultural construction of reality: You take a summer stroll and see someone throw a ball into an open field. Then envision the same scenario, this time with another individual receiving the ball, enfolding it in his catcher's mitt. The mundane action performed by the first person now takes on the character of "pitching" (p. 54).

> Thus, we may commonly identify a baseball game and explore what is required to bring it into existence. But within the traditions of physics or physiology, baseball games do not exist. Thus, whatever we say is forever dependent upon the tradition in which we explore it (p. 59).

Consequently, any explanation remains inherently tied to the specific cultural and historical context in which it is examined. Gergen used such examples to illustrate his point that reality is socio-culturally situated and constructed through the language of that tradition.

That said, Gergen made clear that even though our language frames our reality, it is not that our language is perfect—really quite the opposite. Nouns, participles, and gerunds act to separate, and we end up parsing our world into "entities" (p. xxvi). This carries implications for how we tend to see the world as a conglomeration of separate, individual things instead of a world made up of relationships. Gergen proposes that although nouns make up our language, there is no stand-alone "thing." You may recall Gregory Bateson proposing a similar interconnectedness in our world: Things are always in complex relationships to each other, and to split relationships into "things" is to delude ourselves. However, Bateson did not believe that language, our descriptions and interpretations, creates our realities.

Gergen said this carries over to how we are used to talking about our "self" as a bounded self or bounded being. By atomistically splitting up relationships into entities of "self" and "other," we are not only ignoring the relational aspect, but we are also reinforcing an isolative, individualistic view of human beings that aligns with modern—not postmodern—assumptions. A view of a private self and internal world "invites alienation, loneliness, distrust, hierarchy, competition, and self-doubt" (p. 61). Gergen instead proposes individuals should see themselves as part of relationship webs: mothers to their daughters, sisters to their brothers, etc.

Ironically, Gergen explained, even the idea of a bounded being is a communal construct. It is a sign of the times, so to speak, that the *Cartesian, dualistic* view "of mind and world, subject and object, self and other" (p. xxi) is dominant. Gergen offered a different stance: a postmodern, social constructionist stance that assumes intersubjectivity. What Gergen proposed was an examination of self as fluid, relational, and dialogical.

Gergen erased the static, bounded proposition of a "true" "self." A mother is also a daughter, perhaps a sister, and so on; therefore, "within any relationship, we also *become* somebody" (p. 136). He also discussed the different positions we have such as teacher or learner, contrasting his social constructionist view to a modernist tradition:

> Consider first that within the existing modernist tradition we largely view the student's state of knowledge as an effect for which the educational system is the cause. The system teaches and the student learns: the factory grinds out its product. In this view, we have no easy way of asking about the effects of students on the system. But what if we view the student and the teacher as participants in a relationship? I am not speaking here of a relationship of bounded units, causing each other's movements like so many billiard balls. Rather, they are engaged in a relationship in which they are mutually creating meaning, reason, and value (p. 245).

Gergen highlighted the interconnectedness of human relationships and the capacity for discourse to mutually transform what we know. Like Anderson, he explained that we can engage in transformative dialogue, "which attempts to cross the boundaries of meaning, that locates fissures in the taken-for-granted realities and restores potentials for multibeing, and most importantly, that enables participants to generate a new and more promising domain of shared meaning" (p. 193). Gergen explained that the central focus on the "I" can shift to an emphasis on the collective "we." This shifts our one-way, monological soliloquies and *debates* to two-way *dialogues* where each person learns (technically mutually constructs) something rather than convinces the other.

An invitation to social construction: co-creating the future (4th ed.) (2023)

While the original version was published in 1999, Gergen's fourth edition of his classic text really expands upon the consequences of thinking about knowledge and reality as socially constructed. Gergen's invitation is to consider a social constructionist stance. What possibilities can be opened via such a stance?

Gergen's central opening theme is that what we consider real, rational, good, and so on are products of the social processes we engage in (p. 17). His social constructionist philosophy challenges the empirical view of knowledge that assumes descriptions and explanations should be dictated by an objective reality (p. 19). He called upon his readers to question the supreme authority of the psychiatric discipline and prompted a second look at how certain forms of human activity came to be labeled as "mental illness." He pushed us to consider that what becomes truth is really a numbers game, depending on the consensus of the (in this case, psychiatric and psychological) communities. We are (at least) one step removed from reality; therefore, "*The ways in which we describe and explain the world are the outcomes of relationships*" (p. 20), not observation.

He described how, five decades ago, the prevailing assumption would have been a belief that impartial reporting of facts was indeed achievable and alleged to be proven in scientific, journalistic, and legal contexts (p. 25). They would not have thought twice about the values inherent in the rules or laws nor of the patterns of living and social practices that require closer examination. Gergen made clear his stance that our language, being embedded in our cultural context, carries values with it. Gergen said, "The values of generosity, compassion, love, peace, and indeed life itself, are not intrinsic to human nature. These are terms we have developed in the course of living together" (p. 24). We can shift our conception of knowledge from us being outside observers, documenting the world objectively to an understanding that acknowledges our shaping of our vocabularies, assumptions, and theories about the world and ourselves. Gergen said as we engage in relationships and establish norms and patterns of living, our values unfold. For example, what is "good" depends on our implicit practices. Gergen's philosophy of social construction is an epistemology that accounts for cultural variability, historical evolution, diversity, social agreement, and norms. Thus when we are asked, "What is good?," we reply from our particular social, cultural, and historical contexts.

In this book, Gergen explained how we often think the medical field operates solely on facts and that it neutrally disseminates information or knowledge. Yet this modernist view is an illusion to a social constructionist. From a social constructionist stance, any description takes place in language, so the description itself creates and changes knowledge. To elaborate on his point, Gergen included an example from medical science. Historically, medical textbooks frame women as "baby-makers" (p. 26) which has implications for gender constructs as well as gender roles.

Nevertheless, he emphasized that we should avoid making assumptions that just because scientific assertions are *socially constructed*, they should be *dismissed*. He explained that, just like "death," "cancer" is a social construct; however, most people share the definitions of terms and values—in this case the value of life over death (p. 34): "Within scientific circles, such propositions as 'smoking causes cancer' can be fully verified. And because the values shared within these groups are also shared by large segments of the public, the findings of the sciences can be enormously valuable" (p. 34)

Gergen gave his readers another example of our socially constructed world. He cautioned us to avoid "mistaking the map for the territory" (p. 63). How do we determine the accuracy of a map? What are the consequences on our geographic and historical understandings stemming from the map's construction and acceptance by others?

> While appearing value-neutral, map designers have many choices in depiction, and these choices carry implications for our understanding, of both the world and ourselves. The colors of various areas, the definition of boundaries between regions or countries, and the print size of the labels, for example, can all inform the viewer of the significance, ownership, and prominence of a given nation (p. 64).

Gergen went on to discuss research on discourse and conversation, touching again upon differences in modern versus postmodern thought and alternative, postmodern research methods such as a qualitative research approach called narrative inquiry, autoethnography being one example. In an autoethnography, the researcher is also the participant and person researched. Inside and outside of the research field, his interest was piqued by exploring the relationship between self and other. He offered an invitation to a relational, intersubjective stance of plurality where people can be seen as *multi-beings*, having many voices, roles, and ways of being in the world. He said, "The search for a core self is misguided. In the Western tradition, we have long been taught to 'know thyself.' We are encouraged to find ourselves, to know what we truly want" (p. 121). Contrast this to the alternative position a social constructionist could take:

> The core self is not only misguided but constraining. To be sure, we have habits or conventions that are so comfortable they seem to be expressions of a core. But if we understand these as potential ways of being and not the actual or defining self, we open a space for a more enriched relational life (p. 122).

Related to multi-being is Gergen's explanation of *emerging selves* that result from a dynamic interplay or "dance" of co-action, the term co-action referring to mutual or interactive activities and dialogues between individuals. The idea is that in the process of engaging with others, identities are not fixed but are continually (and mutually) shaped and reshaped. In this view, our sense of self is not static but is continuously evolving through our interactions with others. This aligns with *withness* practice.

Gergen directly addressed social constructionism in psychotherapy, referencing its application in collaborative therapy/C-DP, narrative therapy, and SFBT. His latter chapters are devoted to social constructionism in organizations and governments. I recommend my readers consider his invitation and read his book themselves for more detailed explanations and examples of social constructionism.

PRACTICAL APPLICATION OF GERGEN'S CONCEPTS TO RESEARCH

An anti-traditionalist approach

Gergen's research approach is rooted in social constructionism and *post-positivist* assumptions. Ken and Mary Gergen described social constructionism as an "alternative to a traditional *empiricist* view of science" (Gergen & Gergen, 2011, p. 294). Gergen's critique of empiricist and *positivist* research centered around the nature of the phenomena studied, the measures of the phenomena, and the conclusions about the phenomena. Here is Gergen's own comparison from *An Invitation to Social Construction* (2023):

1. *Positivist:* "Scientists should prevent personal biases from clouding their observations. Research results should not be colored by what they wish or hope to find. Science focuses on what *is* the case, not what *ought to* occur from the researcher's standpoint." (p. 75)
2. *Social constructionist:* "Scientists participate in cultural traditions, and whatever they do as scientists will reflect this participation. All cultural traditions carry certain values or preferred ways of living, and whatever scientists do in the way of research will reflect those traditions. These values enter the research at every point, including the words selected to frame the phenomenon, the research methods, and the description of the results." (p. 76)

For example, even framing a research question in language already introduces preconceived notions and assumptions. The words have historical and cultural "baggage" from their previous use in everyday or scientific communities. Ask yourself how it is that we know what makes a "good research" question in the first place. We were taught. Then ask yourself these important questions: "Who taught us?" and "What was their underlying epistemology?" Give yourself room to question things you have long assumed are "obviously" True.

Qualitative research

Gergen's proclivity for a social constructionist stance led him to have a home in the qualitative research community. Instead of quantitative research's focus on finding truth in numbers, *qualitative research* focuses on finding verisimilitude in stories. It is important to understand that Gergen's critique of traditional research expands beyond research into an epistemological critique. This can be applied across disciplines (see Gergen, 2001).

EXAMPLES OF SOCIAL CONSTRUCTION

Gergen's social constructionist philosophy is founded upon the communal construction of knowledge in context. It takes Truth off its pedestal and contextualizes it as truth; facts become stories, and this process opens space for thorough examination of stories and their effects. Gergen (1985) said, "Regardless of whether we are speaking of scientific fact, canons of logic, foundations of law, or spiritual truths, as we formulate the world, we implicitly favor certain ways of life over others." (p. 268). I include a limited number of examples here. I encourage my readers to seek out Gergen's primary sources should they wish to acquaint themselves with more examples.

Gravity

As a first example, we can explore "gravity." Social constructionism is not making a claim that such a force does not affect us—holding us to the earth and so forth—but that it did not exist *for us* until we named it. "Gravity" came about in a particular cultural, historical, and linguistic context. The naming indicates that it became significant and something we should have a word to talk about.

The word "gravity" was coined by Newton and stems from the Latin "gravitas" which means weight. Instead of a series of random letters, the word gravity came to have a use and thus came to have meaning for us. After naming it, we were able to study it further. Moreover, since the social context around this word transformed over the years, our understanding of what gravity *is* changed over time.

For centuries, it was understood that Earth was the center of the universe (see Ptolemy). Then that was replaced by an understanding that the Earth and other planets orbit the sun (see Copernicus and Kepler). Similarly, "gravity" changed from being a force that keeps *us* from floating off into the ether to being a fundamental force of the *universe*. The language informs us of the socio-cultural influence of an era.

In Newtonian physics, gravity is understood as a force where objects are attracted to each other in relation to their masses and distance. In Einsteinian physics, gravity is the warping of spacetime which results in apparent attraction. These shifting understandings of what gravity *is* across different historical periods underscore the deeply rooted connection between cultural understandings and scientific knowledge.

As a further point, Newtonian physics can still give us accurate measurements in our day-to-day lives and is far more useful in our everyday lives than Einsteinian physics. When high school and college students are taught physics, they are taught Newtonian physics, even if Einsteinian physics is touched upon in more advanced classes. It is far easier to grasp the framework of Newtonian physics. In Newton's Law of Gravitation, gravity is a force that acts between two masses (NASA, 2024, p. 63). Meanwhile, in Einstein's Field Equation, gravity is the curvature of spacetime (NASA, n.d., p. 3). What gravity *is* depends on the context.

In social constructionism, a thing is not naturally a thing, it needs communal agreement. And that is why it can change or even be two contradictory things at once—like gravity. Our understandings shift over time. Therefore, the language, the cultural context of the language, and who is agreeing upon the definition at that time all define what "it" "*is*."

Social constructionists believe we do not have direct access to Reality (i.e., one absolute Reality). Nothing is a thing until it is a thing for us; in other words, nothing has meaning until we give it meaning. And meaning is never one static thing. Meaning is fluid.

Cultural curiosity

Social constructionism is a philosophy that allows for multiple worldviews and thus encourages curiosity rather than pathology, which has implications for how we work with clients. I heard a story from a White American peer in graduate school who was working with a Black American client in her mid-20s. The therapist had written down that the client was engaging in self-harm behavior and noted that the client kept hitting herself on the head. The therapist had written, essentially, that something was wrong with her client and was deliberating over which Diagnostic and Statistical Manual of Mental Disorders (DSM) diagnosis she should consider. If the therapist had provided more space for the client's voice instead of jumping to conclusions, she would have learned that this had nothing to do with self-harm. If she were more aware of Black culture, she would have been conscious of not only hair patting but also the connotations that come with it. For those of you who do not know, hair patting provides scalp relief while preserving your hairstyle. One of the benefits of Gergen's social constructionist beliefs is that it encourages you to ask questions. No matter what cultural backgrounds are at play, the social constructionist therapist does not try to fit the client's worldview within the therapist's; the social constructionist therapist prioritizes the client's worldview and often asks more questions than offers answers. Not believing in one absolute truth, a therapist operating from a social constructionist framework would be immensely curious rather than quick to diagnose.

Gergen talked about how we are quick to jump to conclusions. We often fall into confirmation bias, using professional knowledge to support our clinical hypotheses, which we often justify with professional jargon (Gergen et al., 1996). Gergen questioned the utility and validity of DSM diagnoses through a social constructionist lens (rather than a modernist lens of absolute Truth).

> I find myself increasingly alarmed by the expansion and intensification of diagnosis. Numerous additions to the standardized nomenclature continuously appear in professional writings to the public. Consider, for example, burnout and erotomania. What, we might ask, are the upper limits for classifying people in terms of deficits? (pp. 1–2)

He continued, emphasizing the role of language as constructive in our society:

> As psychological terminologies are disseminated to the public—through classrooms, popular magazines, television and film dramas, and the like—they become available for understanding ourselves and others. They are, after all, the "terms of the experts," and they become languages of choice for understanding or labeling people (including the self) in daily life. Terms such as depression, paranoia, attention deficit disorder, sociopathic, and schizophrenia have become essential entries in the vocabulary of the educated person. Further, when these terms are used to construct the self, they suggest that one should seek professional treatment. In a sense, the development and dissemination of the terminology by the profession acts to create a population of people who will seek professional help. And, as more professionals are required, so is there pressure to increase the vocabulary. Elsewhere (Gergen, 1994) I have called this a "cycle of progressive infirmity" (p. 2).

As professional language trickles down to the public, it affects individual's identity with self and others. As professionals are also members of the public, there is a hermeneutic cycle here as well. Whether we consider our clients as broken, ill, damaged, and so on or as people who are experiencing difficulties associated with the human condition informs us about whether we are operating from a modernist or social constructionist lens.

More examples to consider

Gender identity, race, beauty standards, money, and time are all socially constructed. See if these examples of social constructionist views resonate with your own views:

1. I believe *gender identities*, roles, and expectations are not innate; they are created in societies and vary across culture and time periods.
2. I believe we categorize people into *racial groups* from a cultural more so than biological framework. These categories are created in societies and vary across culture and time periods.
3. I believe *beauty standards* are influenced by the media and popular consensus; these standards are created in societies and vary across culture and time periods.
4. I believe *currency's* value and economic importance is created in societies and varies across culture and time periods.
5. I believe the division of *time* such as by calendar year, time zone, daylight savings time, or even units of measurement are created in societies and vary across culture and time periods.

Gergen is well aware of the controversy surrounding his ideas, and if my reader were to engage in an internal dialogue, it would be most helpful for that dialogue to be, "What are the consequences if I utilize a social constructionist stance?" rather than something like, "Well that's clearly not true." Cultivate self-awareness about how you see the world and look to your language for clues. One's worldview will show through in their language. To borrow song lyrics from Johnny Rivers' (1966) "Secret Agent Man," "Be careful what you say, or you'll give yourself away." Or, as my colleague Paula put it, "Careful, your epistemology is showing."

SUMMARY

Ken Gergen's philosophy is less concerned with the so-called facts of the physical world. Social constructionism attunes to culture, language, and communities. This focus reinforces its clear postmodern foundation because it supports a belief in multiple realities and the communal construction of knowledge.

A modernist might say, "Well, that's your perspective," which can have a patronizing undertone and an implicit message that says, "You're entitled to your opinion even though it's wrong." Alternatively, a social constructionist might say, "Certainly, that fits with your worldview, as best I gather from what you've told me." This latter phrasing supports the other, validating *their* reality, not *the* Reality. Both parties are honored in that latter sentence construction. Notice the second phrasing also uses the language of *fitting*, as though pieces of a puzzle are coming together. It does not claim what is *right*. There is also an implicit asterisk at the end, which holds space for the person to tell them more.

A social constructionist lens is thus conducive to curious, open dialogues rather than close-ended debates. The other's voice is allowed to come through, and, as the dialogue continues, both participants are generating new knowledges together. The participants are not competing for Truth; they are constructing their own truths based on cultural, historical, and temporal societal values. As you will remember from Harlene Anderson's C-DP, generative dialogues are generating knowledge while becoming transformative dialogues, transforming the participants who are shaping and being shaped by the discourse. The relationship creates knowledges, identities, and realities. It may be appropriate to leave modernist readers with one last reminder before this chapter closes:

> The critic wishes a word, "Are you trying to say that nothing exists until there is some kind of relationship? There is no physical world, no mountains, no trees, a sun, and so on? This just seems absurd." In reply, this is not precisely what is being proposed here. We should not conclude that "nothing exists" before the moment of co-action. Whatever exists simply exists. However, in the process of co-action whatever there is takes shape as *something for us*. It comes to be "mountains," "trees," and "sun" in terms of the way we live. Whatever exists does not require distinctions.
>
> *(2009b, p. 37)*

As a social constructionist sees it, our splicing of the world into categories does not help us better understand it. Labels have their purpose and can be useful, but we must remind ourselves to see them as labels, not Truth.

Gergen's provocative philosophy maintains that humans can never achieve a "God's-eye-view" to see, find, discover, or identify *what is really going on* or *what really happened*. As mere humans, we each have our own worldview that is valid. This differs from a perspective that references back to *the Real*. Without access to *the Real*, the concept of perspective falls apart, or at least it is a less useful word for our purposes. Luckily, a social constructionist stance of honoring someone's worldview tends to facilitate respectful and collaborative discussions. While it is not a champion of moral relativism, social constructionism believes all *descriptions* of the world are perhaps better labeled as *stories* since all descriptions take place in a malleable, contextual social framework.

REFLECTIVE QUESTIONS

1. How does social construction fit under postmodernism?
2. In what ways is social constructionism incompatible with modernist philosophy?
3. Can you think of examples of things we take for granted as Real or True that are social constructions?
4. The dominant belief system in psychology and psychotherapy is a modernist epistemology. What are the potential outcomes of that epistemology? What are the potential outcomes of a social constructionist epistemology?
5. How can social constructionism change the psychotherapeutic systems in which we work?

Keywords

Social Constructionism

Social Process

Co-Action

Co-Creation

Tautology

Bounded Self/Being

Cartesian dualism

Monological

Two-Way Dialogues

Generative Discourse

Multi-Beings

Emerging Selves

Post-Positivist

Empiricist

Positivist

Qualitative Research

Ken Gergen's Social Constructionism Post-Test (Inspired by Student Questions)

1. Are social constructionists more culturally competent?
   a. "Culturally competent" itself is a socially constructed term. So we would need to ask the speaker what exactly they meant by this term. However, we can make certain guesses based on our experiences of others using this word and what they might mean. What can be said is that social constructionism is deeply concerned with culture and its influence over the construction of knowledge, and thus the actions we take working from that knowledge. Cultural norms, biases, and prejudices are all taken into consideration.
2. Does social constructionism mean that nothing matters (i.e., nihilism)?
   a. Certainly not. Social constructionism is interested in the meaning-making social processes between individuals. It does not imply that individuals do not have values. Rather, a social constructionist philosophy encourages a discussion of values and beliefs. Social constructionists inquire into context instead of having one definitive answer that is generalized to a whole population.
3. How can social constructionism be taken seriously if it does not believe in facts?
   a. A point of clarity is needed, to say social constructionists do not believe in facts is not entirely true. However, social constructionists do not believe in the absolute objectivity of facts. Using our philosophical capitalization discussed before, they see facts, not Facts. And facts are always grounded in context within the framework from which they were created, studied, and interpreted.
4. Why does Gergen dislike science?
   a. Like Facts, it is not that Gergen does not like science so much as he does not like the reification of Science. Gergen reinforces that science is full of its own traditions, its own biases, and its own prejudices. This does not mean that science is to be discarded. Nietzsche said that "God is dead" to highlight a transition of an era where religion had been replaced by Science in the Enlightenment. Nietzsche's statement encourages us to reevaluate. Similarly,

Gergen seems to push us to reevaluate our taken-for-granted truths. Perhaps we could reorganize them as "helpful assumptions depending on the situation and with limits" rather than take them as "Gospel," so to speak.

5. If I am a therapist, why do I need to know what Gergen thinks about research?

   a. As a social psychologist, Gergen's work includes therapeutic work as well as expands beyond it. It is important to see how social constructionism applies as a philosophy rather than a technique. As a philosophy, when you believe it, you see the world differently and apply that way of thinking across all domains. Additionally, Gergen's work as a researcher moved him away from quantitative research's emphasis on numbers to generalize to qualitative research's emphasis on meaning to resonate. This is a reductive explanation, of course; however, it is useful for the purpose of gaining an initial understanding.

6. What does Gergen mean when he talks about the Bounded Self?

   a. Gergen's use of the term conveys that the self is not a fixed thing, and especially not one "inside" that you get to know "deeper." He views self as shaped and reshaped, just like language. Our identities are created communally, and we know ourselves (understood as fluid) by knowing ourselves with others in our ever-changing social contexts. I am not an "introvert," "extrovert," introverted extrovert," or "extroverted introvert." I am different in different contexts and social situations, engaging in a unique interplay between individual and community.

7. Is co-action simply acting and collaborating with another?

   a. No, co-action refers back to the complex interplay and process of actions and interactions. We engage in verbal and non-verbal language and behaviors that contribute to the construction of realities. Outside of social constructionism, when we talk about action, we usually do not conceptualize it as shifting or changing reality. Co-action in dialogue is a cohesive way of learning via creating.

8. Does the term "multi-being" refer to having different personalities depending on the context?

   a. No, "personality" is a social construct in itself. A social constructionist does not assume they know what "personality" is without asking the person they are communicating with what they mean by that. Furthermore, multi-being refers to our capacity for multiple possibilities for "emerging selves." Instead of a modernist notion of thinking we have seven distinct personalities or a certain number of character traits, Gergen encourages us to see ourselves as forever multitudinous and ever-in-flux. Like Heraclitus' quote, "You cannot step in the same river twice" because the river itself is always flowing and thus changing; we are always growing and changing—not increased by years but by co-action.

9. How can someone believe in multiple realities?

   a. According to a social constructionist, "Reality" is not a thing in itself (that we can *know* at least) but is a social construct itself. What reality means to one person might mean something to another. More importantly, an assumption of one reality takes away from the interpretive and context-dependent aspects social constructionists believe shape our world through our understandings of it. As I heard Gergen tell someone at a conference, when you run into a tree, you certainly do not doubt you ran into a tree. But "tree" did not exist without people to name it thusly. We cannot separate our experience of the world from our interpretation of it.

10. What does this mean? So when I know someone is wrong, I just pretend they are right?
    a. The notions of "right" and "wrong" are socially constructed in cultures and sub-cultures. According to social constructionism, there is no absolute right and wrong, even though most individuals are tied to their values of what they consider right or wrong. No part of social constructionism involves pretending or posturing. Instead, it authentically acknowledges that different people, having, at minimum, different cultural contexts and personal experiences, will have different answers.

11. What is the reason for the excessive quotation marks and unusual capitalization?
    a. Although tedious at times, quotation marks help reinforce that the things we treat as concrete are really ideas, and ideas can change. The unusual capitalization was explained in the Introduction. It is sometimes used in philosophical conversations to distinguish, for example, between a belief in one absolute Truth and multiple truths.

12. I still do not see how social constructionists do not believe in truth or understand their use of truths.
    a. Social constructionists do not reinforce the (to them—erroneous) idea that "truth" can be objective. Social constructionists' use of "truths" highlights that what one sees as true has been influenced by one's language, culture, history, interactions, and the constant shaping and reshaping of interpretation and meaning. Social constructionists are far more likely to be overheard discussing the client's desire to "live their truth," which implies a value of authenticity and acknowledges the uniqueness of the individual while also acknowledging the complex social interplay that contributes to individuals understanding their truth.

KEN GERGEN: PRIMARY SOURCES

Gergen, K. J. (1985). The social constructionist movement in modern psychology. *American Psychologist*, 40(3), 266–275.

Gergen, K. (1998). *When relationships generate realities: Therapeutic communication reconsidered* [Unpublished manuscript]. https://www.swarthmore.edu/sites/default/files/assets/documents/kenneth-gergen/When_Relationships_Generate_Realities.pdf

Gergen, K. J. (2001). *Social construction in context*. Sage.

Gergen, K. J. (2003). *Self and community in the new floating worlds* [Unpublished manuscript]. Swarthmore. https://www.swarthmore.edu/sites/default/files/assets/documents/kenneth-gergen/Self_and_Community_in_the_New_Floating_Worlds.pdf

Gergen, K. J. (2009a). *Relational being: Beyond self and community*. Oxford University Press.

Gergen, K. J. (2009b). Social constructionist movement in modern psychology. *INTERthesis*, 6(1), 299–325.

Gergen, K. J. (2014). From identity to relational politics. In *Postmodern psychologies, societal practice, and political life* (pp. 130–150). Routledge.

Gergen, K. J. (2023). *An introduction to social construction: Co-creating the future* (4th ed., dig. ed.). Sage.

Gergen, K. J., & Gergen, M. M. (2012). Therapeutic communication from a constructionist standpoint. *Discursive Perspectives in Therapeutic Practice*, 65–82.

Gergen, M. M., & Gergen, K. J. (2002). Ethnographic representation as relationship. *Ethnographically Speaking: Autoethnography, Literature, And Aesthetics*, 11–33. https://works.swarthmore.edu/fac-psychology/572

Gergen, M. M., & Gergen, K. J. (2011). Performative social science and psychology. *Historical Social Research*, *36*(4), 291–299.

Gergen, K. J., Hoffman, L., & Anderson, H. (1996). Is diagnosis a disaster: A constructionist trialogue. In F. Kaslow (Ed.), *Relational diagnosis* [draft]. Wiley.

Renowned Sources

Anderson, H. (2011). Reflections on Kenneth Gergen's contributions to family therapy. *Psychological Studies*, *57*(2), 142–149.

Additional References

Haas, D. (2024). *The named generations.* https://geneosity.com/named-generations/

Molière. (2021). *The imaginary invalid* (Trans. C. H. Wall, eBook #9070). Project Gutenberg.

NASA. (n.d.). *Newton's law of gravitation.* https://imagine.gsfc.nasa.gov/observatories/learning/swift/classroom/docs/law_grav_guide.pdf

NASA. (2024). *Exploration brief: Different gravity.* https://www.nasa.gov/wp-content/uploads/2009/07/188961main_Different_Gravity.pdf

Rivers, J. (1966). Secret agent man [song]. On *I know you wanna dance*. Imperial.

The Taos Institute. (2023, November 12). Kenneth J. Gergen, Ph.D. https://www.taosinstitute.net/about-us/people/institute-officers-and-board-of-directors/board-of-directors/kenneth-j-gergen

CHAPTER 3

What ideas from Gergen resonated with Harlene Anderson?

The path to the not-knowing stance

....

Remember, as you read through these chapters, you can always return to the Introduction to refresh your memory on the terms you learned such as positivism, empiricism, constructivism, structuralism, and post-structuralism.

QUESTIONS TO THINK ABOUT

1. What aspects of Ken Gergen's philosophy can be found in Harlene Anderson's and Harry Goolishian's therapeutic approach?
2. Why is it necessary to understand social constructionism to practice C-DP?
3. How might believing in clients' multiple truths change therapeutic outcomes?
4. What is the importance of culture in social constructionism and thus in C-DP?
5. Why is the "not-knowing stance" useful, and what ideas germinate from it?

Chapter 1 introduced collaborative-dialogic practice (C-DP). Chapter 2 covered Ken Gergen's philosophy of social constructionism. Chapter 3 presents the postmodern, social constructionist ideas that resonated with Harlene Anderson and influenced the development of the model she co-founded with Harry Goolishian.

HARLENE ANDERSON'S RESONANCE WITH POSTMODERNISM

Harlene Anderson would have certainly been familiar with *postmodern* thought prior to being introduced to Ken Gergen's social constructionist ideas in 1985; however, since social constructionism is a postmodern philosophy and social constructionism is the foundation of C-DP (Anderson, 2007a), I want to briefly reintroduce postmodernism's

DOI: 10.4324/9781003439349-5

resonance with Anderson. As she described in her major work, *Conversation, Language, and Possibilities: A Postmodern Approach to Therapy*:

> Postmodern thought (often linked with post-structuralism)—usually associated with the writings of philosophers such as Mikhail Bakhtin, Jacques Derrida, Michel Foucault, Jean-Francois Lyotard, Richard Rorty, and Ludwig Wittgenstein—primarily represents a broad challenge to and a cultural shift away from fixed metanarratives, privileged discourses, and universal truths; away from objective reality; away from language as representational; and away from the scientific criterion of knowledge as objective and fixed.
>
> *(Anderson, 1997, pp. 35–36)*

It is widely agreed that postmodernism entails a skepticism toward grand metanarratives and globalized theories, instead creating space for "a plurality of possible descriptions, explanations, and interpretations" (Chenail et al., 2020, p. 419). Metanarratives, overarching narratives or theories which claim to be universal and objective, come under scrutiny. For example, The Big Bang Theory is a metanarrative—a story many believe presents the true facts of our reality and how our universe was created. The Creation Story is another metanarrative—another story many believe presents the true facts about our reality and how our world was created. A belief in one metanarrative will often exclude a belief in another. As evidence of the vast dominance metanarratives can have (even if you do not personally believe them), consider how you likely thought of the Judeo-Christian story of Adam and Eve when I mentioned The Creation Story. Yet many cultures and religions have their own creation narratives about the beginnings of our world. More than an argument for one side, a postmodern attitude is a suspicion of truths that we take for granted (i.e., assume are absolutely true for all people across time). As Anderson put it, "Postmodernism challenges fundamental and legitimizing Truths with a capital T" (2007d, p. 7). The key to shifting from modern to postmodern thought is to view metanarratives as stories or theories rather than truth.

N.B.: neither "metanarrative" nor "narrative" relates to narrative therapy practices in this context.

HARLENE ANDERSON'S RESONANCE WITH KEN GERGEN'S SOCIAL CONSTRUCTIONISM

As you no doubt remember, social constructionism is a postmodern philosophy. When we embrace a postmodern stance, it allows for a belief in multiple realities. The competition for the "right" belief can be eliminated.

Gergen adopted a postmodern stance and made it more specific. By introducing *social constructionism*, Gergen challenged taken-for-granted truths—narratives about knowledge, language, communication, self, and relationships. Regarding modernism, Gergen's philosophy is (1) anti-traditionalist, (2) skeptical of metanarratives, and (3) critical of a positivist or empiricist scientific approach. Regarding postmodernism, Gergen's philosophy is (1) open to multiple ways of knowing, (2) grounded in a sociocultural context, and (3) supportive of inclusive, postmodern research practices. Unlike modernism or even constructivism, Gergen's ideas offered a shift from a bounded being and a traditional focus on the individual to a relational focus on the social being and a focus on relationships and community (Anderson, 2012b).

Knowledge as socially constructed

One of the first assumptions Gergen casts doubt upon is that knowledge exists either "out there" or "inside us." Instead, Gergen proposed that knowledge is created in relationships. Anderson concurred, saying, "I wholeheartedly agree with Gergen. New understandings or 'facts' do not appear spontaneously, nor are they discovered suddenly by an observer. Instead, they evolve from and within "socially negotiated forms of meaning" (Anderson, 1997, p. 14).

According to social constructionism, knowledge is not a *thing*. You cannot give it to someone. Rather than thinking of knowledge as something that can be passed to another, Gergen introduced a way of thinking about knowledge: as something relational and malleable, something fluid that is formed and reformed in language—in dialogue by the people who compose groups, cultures, and societies. Anderson (2001) clearly resonated with this understanding of knowledge, saying, "Knowledge is a by-product of communal relationships rather than an individual possession or product" (Anderson, 2001, p. 345).

When we introduce a postmodern skepticism toward previous understandings of knowledge, we have permission to treat knowledge as narratives rather than a group of facts. Changing "Truth" to "story" does funny things to facts, reality, and knowledge. This allows for more possibilities. Rather than become preoccupied with a pursuit of truth and predictability, one can reorient toward listening, validating, and connecting with the other. We can comment on narratives and how they move us and make us feel and think differently. We do not always have that permissibility in a modernist framework where, often, if you do not see what the framework pushes you to see, you are perceived as unintelligent or deficient in some way. Gergen's ideas about what knowledge *is*, therefore, are associated with freedom from marginalizing modernist practices.

> What we take to be knowledge finds its origins in human relationships. What we believe to be true as opposed to false, objective as opposed to subjective, scientific as opposed to mythological, rational as opposed to irrational, moral as opposed to immoral is brought into being by historically and culturally situated groups of people. Thus, social constructionism first serves an enormous liberating function. It removes the rhetorical power of anyone or any group claiming truth, wisdom, or ethics of universal scope—necessary for all. It is also important to understand that although knowledge claims are socially constructed, this does not render them insignificant. It is to recognize that each tradition, while limited, may offer us options for living together. In this way, social constructionism invites a posture of infinite curiosity.
>
> *(Gergen & Gergen, 2012, pp. 65–66)*

Gergen's social constructionist philosophy encourages us to be curious enough to ask different questions. Instead of, "Is that true?" one might ask, "For whom is that true?" and, "So what?" Gergen's social constructionist ideas place narratives solidly back in their socio-political context—in the communities and societies that made them. Anderson thought "this rejection of global knowledge helped postmodern family therapists focus on the local theories of the family members themselves and to centralize the idea that family members are the best experts on themselves (Chenail et al., 2020, p. 419).

Client expertise and not-knowing

Gergen's ideas naturally reinforce Anderson and Goolishian's *not-knowing* and *non-expert* stances. In 1996, Anderson and Goolishian wrote about a client who had seen several psychologists and felt unheard and unable to tell their story. C-DP's founders wrote:

> Knowing—the delusion of understanding or the security of methodology—can keep us deaf to the unexpected, the unsaid. If we always see and hear things we are accustomed to, we will miss and not see and hear what is different and unique. *Not-knowing* means never understanding too quickly (p. 202).

Aligning with Gergen's understanding of knowledge as fluid and in flux, Anderson and Goolishian saw how the psychologists' act of *knowing too quickly* extinguished the flame of curiosity around this client.

Anderson (2007c) discussed the positive impact of *uncertainty* on her and Goolishian's work as it evolved over time.

> We began to appreciate and value this sense of unpredictability, which, in a strange way, provided feelings of freedom and comfort. We learned that we did not have to know. What we later came to refer to as "not-knowing" liberated us from being content or outcome experts. We did not need to edit clients' stories or realities. We were comfortable that our knowledge was not superior to that of our clients. In turn, our not-knowing perspective allowed an expanded capacity for imagination and creativity. Not-knowing became a pivotal concept and would mark a significant distinction between our and others' ideas about therapy.
>
> *(Anderson, 2007c)*

It is useful to see the not-knowing stance as a position one takes in social constructionism anyway rather than see it as an additional step or technique. Not-knowing is a hesitation toward hypothesizing about Truth. It is a skepticism toward modernist assumptions. Since this skepticism is inherent in social constructionism, and C-DP relies on a social constructionist stance, there is nothing further to "do," except, perhaps, get comfortable with uncertainty (Malinen, 2004).

Pre-knowing and not-knowing

> Dialogue, by its very nature, involves not-knowing and uncertainty. Sincere interest in another necessitates not-knowing the other, their situation, or their

future ahead of time, whether the knowing is in the form of previous experience, theoretical knowledge, or familiarity. Believing that you know the other person, whether from acquaintance with them or as a type of person, can preclude being inquisitive and learning about their uniqueness. Dialogue requires a not-knowing attitude toward its outcome. Because perspectives change and dialogue is inherently transforming, it is impossible to predict, for instance, how a story will be told, the twists and turns its telling may take, or its seemingly final version. Combined, these characteristics distinguish dialogue as a dynamic, generative joint activity and as different from other language activities such as discussion, debate, or chitchat.

(Anderson, 2007b, p. 34)

Forgive my quotations, but to practice Anderson and Goolishian's not-knowing stance is to really question assumptions regarding what "good" "mental health" "treatment" "should" look like. According to Gergen's social constructionist philosophy, knowledge—including knowledge about what therapy *should* look like—is constructed in dialogue, in relationships, in communities, in culture. So there is a narrative about how therapists are *supposed* to be practicing.

Anderson and Goolishian's understanding of not-knowing goes directly against the dominant modernist practice. Yet Gergen's philosophy allowed the co-founders room to consider alternative therapeutic routes. Thus social constructionism provided Anderson and Goolishian with an epistemological platform from which they could better explain their not-knowing position: if mental health practitioners were understanding too quickly, they were not understanding at all. A therapist must respect the client's expertise (Anderson, 2005), lest therapists get stuck in their own ideas about the client and the client's problem rather than curiously listen for the client's ideas about their identity and their problem. Anderson described her experience with a student of hers:

> One young psychiatrist from Nicaragua was talking about the difficult time he was having dealing with uncertainty. He said that, all of a sudden he just decided that there is a lot of certainty in uncertainty. "In being uncertain," he said, "I don't have to know the answer, I don't have to have the best question, I don't have to be the expert doctor. He said that he felt that perspective allowed him to relax and to be much more natural, spontaneous, and present with his clients.
>
> *(Malinen, p. 71)*

Bias and not-knowing

Neither Gergen nor Anderson believed that we should "eliminate" our biases and assumptions because, first, social constructionists believe this process is a delusion, and second, "should" feeds right back into modernism. The postmodern, social constructionist understanding is that we bring our biases and assumptions everywhere we go, and we can work to be attuned to them and manage them. The not-knowing stance helps the therapist avoid confirmation bias and the tendency to put clients into categories—diagnostic or otherwise—instead of seeing them as unique individuals.

Not-knowing is a stance of "not *having to* know" (Anderson, 1997, p. 64). It is not a modernist position of posturing or feigning confusion. It is not an intervention. When you believe in Gergen's social constructionist ideas, it is a natural stance and way of being with others that does not necessitate an expert position. Anderson (2005) emphasized not-knowing as a sincere belief that "over time and through conversation, ideas will change" (p. 497).

In adopting a not-knowing, non-expert stance, space is made for the clients' voices, knowledges, and expertise (Malinen). Consequently, C-DP therapists and clients are equal* conversational partners (well, not quite because of the inherently hierarchical and financially transactional nature of a therapeutic relationship but certainly a significantly lowered hierarchy), and all ideas are up for discussion. Being that social constructionists do not believe in one reigning voice, all understandings, meanings, and possibilities are collaboratively created and recreated through language *between* conversational partners in an "interactive and interpretive process" (Anderson, 1997, p. 72). Thus C-DP is particularly notable for reducing the therapist-client hierarchy, and I do not know of any other mental health model that strives for such a genuinely minimal hierarchy.

MUTUAL INQUIRY: FROM MODERNIST TO POSTMODERNIST PROCESSES

Gergen's interest in research shines through Anderson's work in her use of *mutual inquiry* in therapy. Opposed to the monopolization of modernist research practices, Gergen discussed alternative, less marginalizing research practices. Some qualitative researchers say these alternatives can "put the *human* back in the *human sciences*" (R. Chenail, personal communication, January 14, 2016).

> Particularly within the social sciences, discontent with the alienating conception of scientific research is widespread. Feminist researchers have been especially active in pointing out the manipulative and divisive character of traditional research methods. As a result, adventurous researchers everywhere have begun to create and nurture alternatives. So vibrantly productive are these efforts— often falling under the broad label of *qualitative inquiry*—that the past decade can properly be viewed as a renaissance in research practice. Many of these innovations are specifically dedicated to reducing distance between the scientist and those under study. Or, more properly, the move is away from research *about* others to research *with* them.
>
> *(Gergen, 2009, pp. 235–236)*

Here Gergen continued to provide brief overviews of narrative inquiry (related to stories, not narrative therapy) and autoethnography (i.e., research on the self as a member of a larger culture) as examples of "adventurous" research that appreciates the nuances of the unique individual's experience. Rebellious, postmodern researchers turn away from an "empiricist emphasis on quantifiable behavior" and instead examine "the crucial ingredient of human understanding" (Gergen & Gergen, 2000, para. 6).

Mutual inquiry and reflexivity as a host-guest

As you will recall, Anderson and Gergen are contemporaries who mutually influenced each other. Here, I am highlighting that Anderson's host-guest metaphor can be conceptualized through the same lens as Gergen's mutual inquiry (see Anderson, 2007e). Anderson's focus on the "unconditional hospitality" of a *host-guest*/teacher-learner is reflexive (Anderson, 2007c), just as Gergen's qualitative inquiry where the researcher and participant have a reflexive relationship. Anderson said, "The host's posture, attitude, actions, responses, and tone must communicate to the guest their special importance as a unique human being who is recognized and appreciated" (2012a, p. 15). Anderson's therapeutic position matches Gergen's position on qualitative research, so C-DP relies on the reflexive nature of in-the-moment mutual inquiry.

Mutual inquiry and two-way curiosity

This connects to Anderson's metaphor of a "story ball." Anderson approaches the information clients share as a treasured gift that she politely and graciously inspects while leaving it in the client's hands, looking it over and contemplating it with the client. They hold the story ball together and engage in a mutual process of trying to understand.

Importantly, since social constructionists are not looking to find the Facts or Truth of what happened or is happening, they attend to the detailed stories themselves. Because of this belief in multiple truths and multiple realities, Anderson privileges the client's worldview over her own. There is a philosophical term called "bracketing," which means that you essentially put your own thoughts and beliefs on the back burner so you can fully be in the client's world. This is usually done in phenomenological qualitative research. You can borrow this concept when trying to figure out how you can privilege the client's worldview. Anderson has a related concept called "as-if listening" where you listen as though you were a certain member of the family (2007a).

> The key premise of the "as-if" is that the opportunity for inner and outer dialogue with self and other is enhanced when there is space for speaking and listening: (1) the teller can choose the story to tell and how to tell it and has an unrestricted and protected space to tell it; (2) the listener has an uninterrupted space to listen and time to form his or her responses; (3) there is room for a multiplicity of voices; (4) all hear each voice, none is hidden from the teller; and (5) the teller chooses what invites curiosity and what he or she might like to think or talk about more. There is room for multiple voices and perspectives in storytelling and in reflecting-listening.
>
> *(Anderson, 2007a, p. 38)*

When practicing from the not-knowing stance, you are really doing whatever you can to step into their worldview. How do *they* make meaning of their lives?

You are not trying to tease out Truth. The process, not the outcome, is prioritized. The therapist and client are "co-learners" (2007e) in a dialogical process, so it is about being "in-there-together" (Anderson, 2012a) with the client. Similar to the self-work involved in developing personal and professional cultural competency, there is an error in thinking you have "arrived." The goal is to continuously strive to understand.

Whereas Anderson uses the metaphor of a story ball, I sometimes use the metaphor of a Fabergé egg. The client is offering you a beautiful Fabergé egg, and it is so delicate and precious that you do not want to grab it from them. You simply treasure it, perhaps tracing a pattern with your fingertips as the client holds it for you to see. It is delicate. It is special. It is meaningful. It is beautiful. You are treasuring not only the egg but the experience of them sharing it with you. The interaction is quite moving.

Anderson discussed how two-way curiosity means something more than just listening to the client. She said, "Attentive, careful listening does not guarantee I will hear (understand) what the other person wants me to hear. Listening and hearing require speaking: all are active processes" (2012a, p. 17). With each genuine response, the conversation moves in a certain direction; however, you are not tied to a certain path. Neither are you interested in "proving" something to the client or drawing their attention to what you consider to be an error with a phrase like, "How's that been working out for you?" The curiosity must be genuine and the therapeutic agenda (not "goal") tentative and fluid.

Conversational partners and rethinking hierarchy

Recall *structuralism* and *post-structuralism* from the Introduction. Post-structuralism is moving beyond thinking about structures to thinking about the interconnectedness of communication. Gergen's social constructionist philosophy crosses over post-structuralist ideas such that a social constructionist would not be interested in a hierarchy and roles but on communication and meanings. As Gergen and Gergen (2002) said, "*Traditionally,* we hold individuals to be the units out of which relationships are constructed, thus rendering relationships secondary and synthetic. *Our theoretical work* attempts to reverse this sequence, holding relationship as necessary prior to individual *being*" (p. 27, italics added for emphasis).

Anderson resonated with Gergen's understanding of relationships being formed in and by language rather than by structure. And as Anderson said,

> The thread running through Gergen's contributions then and now is the idea of dynamic social processes. Instead of thinking of the systems that we worked with in therapy as social systems distinguished by predetermined concepts of social role and organization, Goolishian and I thought of the systems of people we worked with (regardless of numbers of people or their relationship to one another) as distinguished by language. In other words, systems, meanings, and understandings are created and exist in language.
>
> *(2012b, p. 143)*

To introduce more etymology to you, let us review the words *context*, *construct*, and *converse*. These words are based on the common Latin root *con*, meaning "with" or "together." CONtext means "to weave together," CONstruct means "to build together," and CONverse means "to live or have dealings together." Gergen and Anderson's shared epistemology is that conversations (i.e., "to have dealings together") construct (i.e., "build together") realities. The context of stories is the "weaving together" of stories; therefore, it is impossible to extract stories out of context, and it is impossible to build together without sharing in the co-construction of meanings. As Ken Gergen (2023) said,

> The conversation metaphor is a congenial companion for social construction-ists, as it is largely in conversation that worlds of meaning are co-created. How participants define the organization, themselves, and their relationship, along with the value of their activities depends on the conversations in which they participate. Rather than parts of a machine, people can become *conversational partners* (pp. 211–212).

(In the quote above, Gergen used Anderson's term "conversational partner" which is a clear demonstration of their mutual influence). If a therapist conducts a C-DP session successfully, they become a conversational partner. The conversational partners engage in what Gergen calls "co-action" (Gergen, 2009). "As conversational partners, we continually coordinate our actions as we respond with and thus affect each other" (Anderson, 2012a, p. 20).

Can you see why I said the hierarchy is lowered to be more egalitarian in C-DP and why Anderson described it as an "in-there-together" process? If not, perhaps another example may help. Can you see how laughing *with* someone is different than laughing *at* them? Anderson built C-DP around talking with someone rather than at them. There are shared, special moments in an inside joke, and there are shared special moments in a C-DP conversation where *withness* is prioritized. The hierarchy of "therapist-client" is inherent, but it is not used as a tool or intensified as an intervention. In applying Anderson's not-knowing stance, you employ a different understanding of hierarchy than the modernist understanding you were likely taught in school. Again, Anderson's not-knowing, non-expert stance emphasizes the client as the expert rather than the therapist: "The expertise of the therapist is rooted in, and defined by, capacity to risk participation in dialogue and *con*versation, and to risk changing" (Anderson, 2005, p. 498, italics added for emphasis).

Withness and mutual transformation

Anderson places importance upon the idea that the therapist is changed in therapy, which is often revelatory for new therapists. This clearly aligns with a social construc-tionist stance; whereas a modernist would say you are "too close" to your client or perhaps "not differentiated enough" if you are moved by them. In general systems and cybernetic systems theories, therapists are seen as agents of change. Within Gergen's social constructionist framework, C-DP therapists see themselves as participants in transformative dialogue. C-D practitioners seek out opportunities to practice the art of "withness."

Because of this unique interaction of engagement between therapist and client, both parties are, ideally, moved by the experience. Mutual transformation can take place. As Anderson said, "Each person is under the influence of the other; hence, each is "at-risk" for change. The process is not a one-sided, unilateral therapist-driven activity, nor is a therapist merely passive and receptive" (Anderson, 2012a, p. 20). Do not assume "at-risk" above is just about the clients; Anderson used derivatives of the phrase "at-risk for change" to emphasize what therapists are faced with in C-DP. Because the therapist is collaborating so closely with the client in a not-knowing stance, they are in the therapeutic space with them; there is little chance they will not be transformed by this experience if it is genuine.

Not-knowing and being public

In C-DP, you must be in the client's world, in their truth, and in their language with them. You are not persuading, dissuading, assigning homework, and so on. You are meeting them where they are, and you will construct something new together through dialogue. There should not be a battle between a client's truth and the assumed truth. Their truth *is* their truth.

Being public is a part of the process of adopting a not-knowing stance during a therapy session. It is a way for you to speak aloud thoughts that might otherwise spiral into an internal monologue that would take you out of their story. It can be as simple as, "Hold on one second, I have to get my thoughts straight. Did you say, ...?" This is a way of checking in, being polite, and being public before that pesky thought gets in the way of the entire conversation. It also avoids the modernist temptations like assuming your client is lying to you and spending the rest of the session trying to be a detective instead of a therapist.

SUMMARY

Harlene Anderson and Harry Goolishian first came across Ken Gergen's written works in the 1980s. Unfortunately, Goolishian passed away in 1991, but Gergen and Anderson have been able to maintain a long-term professional relationship of mutual influence and reflexivity. They will often use the same or similar language. It is interesting to see how they have arrived at the same therapeutic conclusions, having initially approached it from different starting points: one from epistemology to therapy and the other from therapy to epistemology.

Gergen's social constructionism is fundamental to the practice of C-DP. Everything is based around understanding and believing in social constructionist ideas before refining the art of therapy. The not-knowing stance is not a technique but fits within the framework of understanding that the client is the expert, that client and therapist are on a mutual journey, and that therapy is a reflexive process where meanings and realities are constructed in language. Instead of trying to practice how to "do" the not-knowing stance, consider whether the philosophy aligns with your personal beliefs. If not, continue your search for a model whose epistemology fits with your own.

REFLECTIVE QUESTIONS

1. How does qualitative inquiry relate to mutual inquiry?
2. How does mutual inquiry relate to conversational partners?
3. Why is post-structuralism relevant to seeing dialogue as constructive?
4. How is "being public" relevant to mutual transformation?

Keywords

Postmodernism

Metanarratives

Social Constructionism

Not-Knowing Stance

Client Expertise

Mutual Inquiry

Host-Guest

Conversational Partners

Structuralism

Post-Structuralism

Transformative Dialogue

Being Public

The Not-Knowing Stance Post-Test (Inspired by Student Questions)

1. Is there any order or procedure for the structure of sessions and when to use the not-knowing stance like during an intake or family history?
   a. No, there are no procedural steps in C-DP, and you and the client mutually agree upon what is discussed each session. Each session is inimitable, as each relies on the withness practices. The stance is constant because it is your consistent viewpoint.
2. If you are practicing the not-knowing stance, what do you do if you disagree with a client?
   a. The not-knowing stance does not mean you forget everything. You are free to disagree with your client. The main thing is how you bring it up. If you are being public and bring it up as "just an idea," that is something that you and the client can work on collaboratively. A tentative position goes a long way (see Anderson, 2007e).
3. How do I know that I am doing anything helpful for the client?
   a. Although some mistake it for being passive, the not-knowing stance is an active process, requiring skill to stay in-the-moment and avoid jumping to conclusions. As far as helpfulness goes, C-D therapists check in with their clients often to make sure therapy is useful for them.
4. How can I adopt a not-knowing stance when I know sessions need to achieve a certain goal?
   a. The idea that you need to achieve a certain goal is a modernist one. Not to say that a C-D therapist has no sense of direction, but that direction, that agenda, is fluid. Remember that C-D practitioners believe problems can be dis-solved in language, in the process of the transformative dialogue.

5. The not-knowing stance seems to imply a certain lack of initiative on the part of the therapist. What do you do when clients directly ask you to tell them what to do?

   a. When you say, "a lack of initiative" it indicates that you have a pre-understanding of what therapy should look like. We all enter the therapy room with certain expectations and pre-conceived notions, and this is why it is important to lay the groundwork for having conversations with your client where you let them know this will be unlike conversations that they may have seen in the media or had with a prior therapist. It is a perfect opportunity for you to practice being public.

6. What is the most important thing to know about social constructionism and the not-knowing stance?

   a. That social constructionism is a philosophy, a group of ideas that you believe in. It is most important to remember that it is a belief that truths, realities, and meanings are co-*con*-structed and collaboratively re*con*structed. The not-knowing stance is a position you adopt while within the social constructionist philosophy. The not-knowing stance lies seamlessly within Gergen's social constructionism.

7. How do you learn to be a C-D practitioner?

   a. I believe this is best answered by Anderson herself: "I do not think that I can teach, train, or instruct a therapist how to be a collaborative/conversational therapist or to have the philosophical stance. I can, however, provide a dialogic space and process for being in relationship and conversation with each other in which learning occurs for all…. Letting go of 'thinking and acting like a therapist' is at the heart" (Anderson, 2007a, p. 33).

HARLENE ANDERSON: PRIMARY SOURCES

Anderson, H. (1997). *Conversation, language, and possibilities: A postmodern approach to therapy.* Basic Books.

Anderson, H. (2001). Postmodern collaborative and person-centered therapies: What would Carl Rogers say? *Journal of Family Therapy, 23,* 339–360.

Anderson, H. (2005). Myths about "not-knowing". *Family Process, 44*(4), 497–504.

Anderson, H. (2007a). Creating a space for a generative community. In H. Anderson & P. Jensen (Eds.), *Innovations in the reflecting process* (pp. 33–45, dig. ed.). Routledge.

Anderson, H. (2007b). Dialogue: People creating meaning with each other and finding ways to go on. In H. Anderson & D. Gehart (Eds.), *Collaborative therapy: Relationships and conversations that make a difference* (pp. 33–42, dig. ed.). Routledge.

Anderson, H. (2007c). Historical influences. In H. Anderson & D. Gehart (Eds.), *Collaborative therapy: Relationships and conversations that make a difference* (pp. 21–32, dig. ed.). Routledge.

Anderson, H. (2007d). Postmodern umbrella: Language and knowledge as relational and generative and inherently transforming. In H. Anderson & D. Gehart (Eds.), *Collaborative therapy: Relationships and conversations that make a difference* (pp. 7–20, dig. ed.). Routledge.

Anderson, H. (2007e). The heart and spirit of collaborative therapy: The philosophical stance—"A way of being" in relationship and conversation. In H. Anderson & D. Gehart (Eds.), *Collaborative therapy: Relationships and conversations that make a difference* (pp. 43–59, dig. ed.). Routledge.

Anderson, H. (2012a). Collaborative relationships and dialogic conversations: Ideas for a relationally responsive practice. *Family Process*, *51*, 8–24.

Anderson, H. (2012b). Reflections on Kenneth Gergen's contributions to family therapy. *Psychological Studies*, *57*(2), 142–149.

Ken Gergen: Primary Sources

Gergen, K. (2009). *Relational being: Beyond self and community*. Oxford University Press.

Gergen, K. J. (2023). *An introduction to social construction: Co-creating the future* (4th ed., dig. ed.). Sage.

Gergen, K. J., & Gergen, M. M. (2012). Therapeutic communication from a constructionist standpoint. *Discursive Perspectives in Therapeutic Practice*, 65–82.

Gergen, M. M., & Gergen, K. J. (2000). *Qualitative inquiry: Tensions and transformations* [Unpublished manuscript]. https://www.swarthmore.edu/sites/default/files/assets/documents/kenneth-gergen/Qualitative_Inquiry_Tensions_and_Transformations.pdf

Gergen, M. M., & Gergen, K. J. (2002). Ethnographic representation as relationship. *Ethnographically Speaking: Autoethnography, Literature, and Aesthetics*, 11–33. https://works.swarthmore.edu/fac-psychology/572

Renowned Source

Malinen, T. (2004). The wisdom of not-knowing: A conversation with Harlene Anderson. *Journal of Systemic Therapies*, *23*(2), 68–77.

Additional Reference

Chenail, R. J., Reiter, M. D., Torres-Gregory, M., & Ilic, D. (2020). Postmodern family therapy. *The Handbook of Systemic Family Therapy*, *1*, 417–442.

PART III

Narrative Therapy

CHAPTER 4

An introduction to narrative therapy

....

> Remember, as you read through these chapters, you can always return to the Introduction to refresh your memory on the terms you learned such as positivism, empiricism, structuralism, post-structuralism, Cartesian dualism, and social constructionism.

QUESTIONS TO THINK ABOUT

1. What is the meaning and composition of a story? Of therapy?
2. How does a narrative therapist see the client differently through this model's lens?
3. Is narrative therapy a social constructionist model?
4. What is a decentered position and why is this important?
5. According to White, what role does the DSM play in our daily lives?
6. How does a narrative therapist re-author?

Michael White was an Australian social worker and family therapist who, along with New Zealander David Epston, founded a postmodern therapy practice called *narrative therapy* in the early 1980s (Anderson, 2015). Narrative therapy explores the meanings clients make of their life stories and the ways in which society contributes to the construction of personal identities (White & Epston, 1990). Culture is not an afterthought in narrative therapy; it is built within the model. Unlike other therapy models, narrative therapy has a thread of social justice woven throughout, and it is in many ways compatible with feminist, queer, and postcolonial studies (Madigan, 2019), "decolonizing areas of life from Western psychological understandings" (Denborough, 2019, p. 19).

According to one of White's mentees, Stephen Madigan, narrative therapy was the first therapy model that involved an active analysis of power relations (2019, p. 19). White and Epston helped clients reevaluate societal norms, seeing them anew as stories

DOI: 10.4324/9781003439349-7

they could opt in or out of rather than rules they were mandated to follow. For an example, we can look to White's (1991) words himself.

> I asked specifically about how the problems had been influencing the client's thoughts about *herself*: What did *she* believe these problems reflected about her as a parent? Was the havoc that the view of *failure*, and its associated guilt, was wreaking in the client's life and her relationships *acceptable* to her? Or would she feel more comfortable if she broke her life and her relationships *free of the tyranny* of this view and its associated guilt?
>
> *(pp. 21–22, italics added for emphasis)*

Freedom and choice are recurring themes in White's work, as is knowledge and power. These are discussed more fully in the next chapters which help you understand Michel Foucault's influence on White and the development of narrative therapy.

Narrative therapy challenges *positivist* assumptions because it believes reality is beyond measure. It challenges *empiricist* assumptions because it assumes reality is beyond what we can see, hear, smell, taste, or feel. Therefore, narrative therapy, like collaborative-dialogic practice (C-DP), challenges the idea that we can measure Reality or get "closer" to Reality via the imagined aid of our five senses or application of the scientific method.

This may be contrasted against models that rely on empirical findings and modernist research-based interventions. To varying degrees, Applied Behavior Analysis (ABA), Cognitive Behavioral Therapy (CBT), and The Gottman Method are certainly examples of modern models with the label "evidence-based" that insurance companies seem to value so highly. Yet, like the other postmodern models, narrative therapy holds a belief that things are more than they appear—and discourses cannot be ignored! So just because it was not built upon modernist research does not imply a lack of research to support its efficacy.

THE ADVENTUROUS SPIRIT OF THE CO-FOUNDERS

White and Epston were friends and colleagues whose lives and ideas influenced one another's imaginations "down the rabbit hole" of narrative therapy (see Marsten et al., 2016). These therapists brought their personal lives and passions into the development of narrative therapy. Their therapy blended serious work with their avant-garde "spirit of adventure" (White & Epston, 1992, p. 9, as cited in Malinen et al., 2012, p. xvi).

White was enamored with jazz music and readers can see examples of White using jazz as a metaphor to describe a therapist developing their skill or expertise over time. Epston talked about how "learning the scales precedes learning how to improvise" (Epston et al., 2019, p. 5). White and Epston encouraged therapists to be spontaneous and improvisational, while maintaining meticulous focus on their language in the therapeutic practice.

Epston was interested in cultural anthropology and artifacts, which no doubt influenced his work. Epston compiled "archives" of artwork, audio recordings, and letters that supported the client and countered the problem (Madigan & Epston, 1995, p. 3). He decided to turn his case notes into verbatim transcripts of the client's words rather than employ an expert-stance report which, to a postmodern eye, would be more befitting of the natural sciences than the human sciences (Madigan, 2019). Epston and White would celebrate client's progress "by encouraging awards, diplomas, and parties" (p. 14).

You will no doubt come across video recordings of White with a happy smirk on his face, likely while making puns. White had a playful approach to therapy and education which we can see shine through his workshops. For instance, when a cell phone interrupted a workshop conference, he told the attendees they could decide whether they wanted their phones on or off, but if they chose to leave them on, they had to commit to singing along to the ringtone if it rang (Winslade & Hedtke, 2008).

White and Epston proved you can talk about serious issues with a lighthearted, rebellious spirit often associated with postmodernism (see Freeman et al., 1997). Narrative therapy rejects taken-for-granted assumptions and modernist norms that dictate what therapy "should" look like. The founders ethically used humor throughout their work.

NARRATIVE THERAPY: MOVING BEYOND GENERAL SYSTEMS THEORY AND CYBERNETICS

Like C-DP, narrative therapy is a profoundly different approach compared to modernist mental health approaches. Narrative practitioners Vetere and Dowling (2016) acknowledged the helpfulness of the introduction of family therapy's general systems theory in shifting a historically individualist psychological conceptualization of problems into *a systemic, relational* conceptualization of problems in context. However, narrative therapy evolved even further *beyond* general systems theory/cybernetics theory—adopted by the Mental Research Institute (MRI; 1950s), structural family therapy (1960s), and The Milan Team (1970s) (Boston, 2018)—by incorporating the social science's "cultural turn" (Rustin & Rustin, 2016, p. 27) during the 1970s and 1980s (p. 30) which challenged the categorizations practiced in *structuralism.*

The philosophical movement of structuralism, as you will recall from the Introduction, holds that systems themselves create organizing roles in families, establishments, and cultures. As narrative therapy practitioners Rustin and Rustin said, "The structuralists, following the cultural anthropologist Claude Levi-Strauss, held (in the "strong" version of the rationalist program) that cultures were universally structured by means of binary classifications" (p. 30).

You will also recall that *post-structuralism* is a philosophy that critiques structuralism as reductive and rejects structuralist attempts at any universalization of human experience. Like C-DP, narrative therapy borrows from post-structuralist philosophy, believing "it is useful to focus on contextualized meaning-making rather than on universal truths or an all-encompassing reality" (Combs & Freedman, 2012, p. 1036).

Narrative therapy, in simple terms, got rid of the *system* (in the traditional, modernist family therapy sense) but kept the *relational* in "systemic, relational family therapy." Narrative therapy critiques thinking about the family as a "rigid arrangement of people" in systems (Combs & Freedman, 1996, p. 1). Instead, narrative therapy adopts social constructionism's focus on people's stories and communal meaning-making. In social constructionism, "words and language derive meaning from the relational, emotional contexts in which they are used" (Dowling & Vetere, p. 5).

RECALLING NEW KNOWLEDGES AND APPLYING
THEM IN NARRATIVE THERAPY

I would like to take a pause here to reinforce what I assume for many of my readers composes new knowledges ("knowledges" is intentionally pluralized). You may have noticed the evolutionary path of narrative therapy is parallel to that of C-DP. It moved from cybernetic and general systems theory metaphors to seeing the world as socially constructed in discourse. Since the epistemology of social constructionism is central to narrative practice, just as it is to C-DP, I want to review what you have already learned.

Postmodernism is a philosophical belief in multiple realities and truths. Postmodernists challenge a belief in an objective reality or Truth. In the absence of Truth, narrative therapists, being postmodern, focus on exploring clients' truths (lowercase "t").

Social constructionism is a philosophy that upholds our worldviews are socially created through language and discourse. Social constructionists challenge a belief in absolute Knowledge, Reality, and Meaning. Instead, narrative therapists focus on exploring clients' knowledges (lowercase "k"), realities (lowercase "r"), and meanings (lowercase "m").

As explained earlier, the unusual capitalization found in this book is meant to help distinguish whether the words are being used in an objective manner. Capital letters are an indication of objectivity or a universal idea. This style can be found in philosophical literature as well as alternative family therapy resources on postmodern practices (e.g., Korman et al., 2020).

NARRATIVE THERAPY: THE LABEL OF SOCIAL CONSTRUCTIONISM

As mentioned, narrative therapy is postmodern, operating based on a belief in multiple truths and multiple realities. It challenges positivist and empiricist assumptions about truth and knowledge. Narrative therapy practices are also influenced by poststructuralism, particularly as it relates to identity (Marsten et al., 2016; White, 2005) and highlight context and communication. Narrative therapy practices are also social constructionist (Combs & Freedman, 1996), emphasizing the interplay of social relationships, language, and culture in forming our worldviews.

Co-founder David Epston and his colleagues referenced Gergen's social constructionist views in their co-authored book (2016). Narrative therapists Gene Combs and Jill Freedman wrote an exceptional book (1996) entitled *Narrative Therapy: The Social Construction of Preferred Realities*, which was quite literally endorsed by White—as you can read on the back cover. Despite these and other countless instances of narrative therapy being understood and accepted as a social constructionist model, it is my belief that White was not wholly comfortable using the term social constructionist to describe his narrative practices (see Malinen et al., 2012). I do not want to muddy the waters, but I wish to be candid.

Before the deaths of Tom Andersen in 2007 and Michael White in 2008, White engaged in a dialogue with Harlene Anderson and Tom Andersen where they were inviting White to discuss his model within the realm of social constructionism, White explained his thoughts on the subject:

> One constructivist position is that everything is constructed in language, and that we only have constructions. My own approach is more Foucauldian. Foucault

argues that constructions of knowledge are always associated with practices of living, and the two are not the same. These constructions and practices are in a relationship of mutual dependency, but they are not one and the same thing. There are constructs of the world and there are practices of living—practices of the self and practices of relationship—which are intimately linked to those constructs.

(White, 2012, p. 144)

The next two chapters address Foucault's undeniable influence on White. Here, I would like to share my interpretation of White's view without going into too much detail about Foucault at this time.

In line with postmodernism's skepticism toward metanarratives, White and Epston were certainly skeptical of labels and made it a point to avoid labeling whenever possible. In their co-authored book, they declared: "We do not identify with any particular 'school' of family therapy, and we believe that such a naming would only subtract from our freedom to explore various ideas and practices" (White & Epston, 1990, p. 9). Since at least 1990, we can see evidence of narrative therapy practices eschewing labels and categorization. This explains why White would be hesitant to label his model as a social constructionist.

At the same time, White and Epston's model postulates that (1) individuals exist relationally in communities, (2) knowledge is communally constructed, and (3) discourse is constructive of our realities. As a further point, White also said, "An objective knowledge of the world is not possible, and knowledges are actually generated in particular discursive fields" (White, 1993, p. 125, as cited in Ilic, p. 86). Although White may have been hesitant to apply the label, these are certainly social constructionist ideas. This is why narrative therapy is known as a social constructionist family therapy model—just like the other two postmodern family therapy models addressed in this book.

As additional support for my assertion, even Epston cites social constructionist philosopher Ken Gergen in a book co-written with narrative therapists David Marsten and Laurie Markham where they discussed the importance of our social world in constructing how we see ourselves and how we see ourselves in relation to others.

Given that meaning is negotiated relationally, how we come to know ourselves is more a consequence of social engagement than the result of private meditation. The notion that self-esteem is found *within* may be alluring. But hope of pinning it down, once and for all, no more reliable than the sighting of a Cheshire Cat in the branches of a tree—here one moment and gone the next. Ultimately, it is in the context of relationships that we know ourselves as more or less capable.

(Marsten et al., 2016, p. 108, italics
added for emphasis)

I wish to summarize this point that narrative therapy is a social constructionist family therapy model. Social constructionism is a view that knowledge is constructed socially, in discourse, set within a particular cultural and historical context. This certainly applies to narrative therapy. However, it is well known that White had discomfort around any "-ism," so it is not surprising that White would hesitate to adopt this label, even if Epston seemed more comfortable with it.

White likely objected to the label because it brought his model more into Gergen's philosophy than Foucault's philosophy, and White was so aligned with Foucauldian ideas and values that he could not discard them, even temporarily. "[Narrative practitioner] Jim Duvall often said that White did not practice a therapeutic 'brand;' he practiced 'Michael White therapy'" (Duvall & Béres, p. 14). During the conversation with Harlene Anderson and Tom Andersen, both respected White's wishes to avoid the label.

ROLE OF THE THERAPIST

White adopted a consultative stance, not an expert stance. White was aware of the commonplace duplicity of therapists who, on the one hand, feigned genuine curiosity with a "tell me more" statement and, on the other hand, had already drawn definitive conclusions about the problem, the client, and how the client *should* solve the problem. White noticed and fully appreciated the inherent power dynamics in being an intern or licensed mental health professional with a client. Therefore, White took extra care to empower clients in his therapeutic work while taking responsibility for therapists' culpability in co-authoring clients' stories (2007).

Adoption of a decentered yet influential position

Like jazz, narrative therapy features an improvisational nature over structure and a performer (client) over composer (therapist). Unlike so many modernist founders that preceded them, White and Epston had the client—not the therapist—take center stage. White and Epston approached clients with humility. White's term of "interviews" emphasizes the nature of narrative work as a consultation rather than a session where the so-called "patients" are "fixed" (White, 2007).

Placing the client and their story at the center of therapy was referred to as the therapist taking a *"decentered"* (because the client is at the center) and *"influential"* (because a therapist can never *not* be influential) position (Ilic, 2017; Wand & Pepe, 2023; White & Morgan, 2006). Whereas a centered, influential position creates an expert therapist who intervenes, a decentered, influential position creates a non-expert therapist who redirects. Morgan (2002) said narrative therapists would "decline invitations to be the expert" (p. 86).

> A centered therapeutic position places the therapist at the center of the therapeutic interaction, whereas a decentered therapeutic position places the client(s) at the center of the therapeutic interaction. For example, a decentered therapeutic position is one in which "the therapist is not the author of people's positions on the problems and predicaments of their lives" (White, 2007, p. 39). Rather, the client's voice is privileged over the therapist's expert knowledge.
>
> *(Ilic, 2017, p. 5)*

By embracing a decentered yet influential position, narrative therapists could do more dynamic work. Instead of carrying out psychological evaluations that sought to identify the so-called dysfunctions, narrative therapists became story-focused. The client becomes the "author-ity" (Crocket 1999, 2004, as cited in Pare, 2012, p. 23). If a therapist believes stories and identities are malleable, changing these stories can restore hope to clients.

Like C-DP, a narrative therapist adopts a curious, non-hierarchical, non-expert, non-pathologizing, and not-knowing stance. However, whereas a C-DP therapist may take a position that appears more like a conversation between friends, a narrative therapist will take a decentered, influential position that is relatively more structured. A narrative therapist is "tuning their ear" (Hibel & polanco, 2010) for discourses and "listening for" dominant discourses and questioning them.

A RADICAL VIEW OF THE CLIENT: THE PERSON IS NOT THE PROBLEM

Returning to the Marsten et al. (2016) excerpt above, we see the importance of relational context. One of narrative therapy's key understandings is the belief that clients exist in relation to problems, but they are not defined by them (White, 1991). In other words, narrative therapy focuses on people being *in relation* to a problem rather than *being* the problem (Morgan, 2002). Thus it is known for its popular saying, "The person is not the problem; the problem is the problem" (Madigan, 2019, p. xxv).

According to White (2007), people often feel that something is wrong with them when they encounter one of life's many difficulties.

> Many people who seek therapy believe that the problems of their lives are a reflection of their own identity, or the identity of others, or a reflection of the identity of their relationships. This sort of understanding shapes their efforts to resolve problems, and unfortunately these efforts invariably have the effect of exacerbating the problems. In turn, this leads people to even more solidly believe that the problems of their lives are a reflection of certain "truths" about their nature and their character, about the nature and character of others, or about the nature and character of their relationships. In short, people come to believe that their problems are internal to their self or the selves of others—that they or others are in fact, the problem (p. 9).

Separating the person from the problem, White and Epston changed how practitioners conceptualized the identified patient (IP) and their problematic situation, which had the effect of highlighting clients' self-agency while valuing each client's unique story. Illustratively, White adopted the language of therapeutic "interviews" instead of "sessions." He also tended to use a longer phrase such as "someone who was interviewed" instead of "patient" or even "client" (see Combs & Freedman, 2012) or to simply use the person's name (see White, 2007). By viewing individuals as people limited by societal norms and stories that did not fit for them, White and Epston (1990) saw a way therapists could move away from modernist psychological traditions of categorizing people by their problems or the modernist general systems' theory tradition of problems "serving a function" in a family system (Haley, 2010).

Marsten et al. implied that traditional modernist approaches put the therapist in a paternalistic position (2016), whereas narrative therapy adopted a non-expert stance. White and Epston did not see clients as less than, internally deficient, or damaged. Indeed, narrative therapy does not perpetuate an internal, individualistic view of the self like our "poster child" of the Enlightenment, René Descartes (Madigan). Cartesian dualism, along with modern liberal theory, is responsible for people thinking they are "internal miners"—as White joked—"digging deep to get in touch with their [personal] resources" (as cited in Denborough, 2019, p. 14).

Narrative therapy adopts a view that people's lives are multi-storied; we come to know ourselves from our relationships with others rather than something that allegedly lies within us. Stories are not just some*thing* we share. Stories *create* and dictate our actions: "Although people live and construct stories about their lives and relationships, stories also live through and construct people's lives and relationships" (Madigan, p. 71). Can we know we are funny without another person to laugh? Can we know we are funn*ier* without having multiple others to whom we can compare? If we tell ourselves and others, "I am the funny one; Laura is the smart one," how much does this story affect the decisions we will make in the future?

White and Epston believed clients' problems were tied to limiting stories, influenced by relationships and societal norms and standards. The problem story narrows a client's experience of themselves and others. Clients' presenting problems are part of an apocryphal narrative in which the problem is maintained by tacit or overt agreement within a limiting story. As the founders saw it, the problem lingered because the clients' narratives storied the problem as intractable. White and Epston were interested in developing a counter-narrative. But they first needed to understand "how persons organized their lives around specific meanings and, in so doing, inadvertently contributed to the 'survival' of, as well as the 'career' of, the problem" (White & Epston, p. 3).

STORYTELLING AND NARRATIVES

White was influenced by many fields, including psychology, literary theory, and anthropology (White, 2011). The work of constructivist Jerome Bruner underlies narrative therapy insofar as he thought words—stories—shape our meaning-making and, thus, our lived experiences (Marsten et al., 2016). Bruner saw humans as storytelling beings and believed we cannot help but create stories to make sense of our world. He highlighted that we are the authors of our stories, not just the main characters. Aligning with White's Cartesian critique, Bruner said, "It is through narrative that we create and recreate selfhood, that self is a product of our telling and not some essence to be delved for in the recesses of subjectivity" (as cited in Ilic, p. 88).

This usage of the word "narrative" in the quotation above ties into how we usually think about stories: chronologically with a beginning, middle, and end and with characters and plotlines. White, on the one hand, accepted this usage while, on the other hand, made it something more by also incorporating Foucauldian ideas, thereby creating narrative therapy as we have come to know it. When White engaged with Foucauldian ideas (discussed in the next chapter), "narrative" took on a meaning beyond storytelling. To understand narrative in this secondary way, you must stop thinking about narratives as mere storylines and instead think about them as discourses.

DISCOURSES AND NARRATIVES

Discourses refer to certain types of narratives maintained by complex social dynamics within society involving power, knowledge, and truth. A discourse is a story told by society that a lot of people agree with such that it ends up transforming how we think about knowledge as well as power relations. Whereas discourses in C-DP are related to ideas about social constructionism (i.e., Gergen), discourses in narrative therapy may include more overtly political understandings about power (i.e., Foucault). Although more similar than dissimilar, these two are slightly at odds because Foucault had an understanding about the ways in which power-knowledge operates, making it a dash more modern. A belief in the way that power "truly" operates increases certainty about "the effects" of "power." The more certainty we have that "this is the way it is," the less skeptical we are and the less postmodern we are. Still, narrative therapists certainly do not believe in globalizing truths.

In the absence of absolute truth, we can analyze *dominant discourses*, predominant or reigning narratives that are the result of practices of power. Narrative therapy assumes individuals are shaped by discourses: those of larger society, those of sub-cultures, and those of sub-communities and families. Dominant discourses, sometimes masquerading as Truth, can classify ideas and behaviors into "right" and "wrong" and people into categories. White (1991) pointedly asked, "What is the origin of these discourses or narratives that are constitutive of persons' lives?" (p. 28). Answering his own question, he said, "Our culturally available and appropriate stories about personhood and about relationships have been historically constructed and negotiated in communities of persons" (p. 28).

White believed dominant discourses can have a devastating effect on individuals and families. They inherently involve a reductive classification of multifaceted individuals within a complex social, political, and cultural web. We are so surrounded by and immersed in these discourses that it can be difficult to think in ways that challenge these ideas.

You yourself have likely been guilty at one point or another of thinking people "are" *this* or *that*, good or bad, happy or depressed, healthy or unhealthy, and so on. Our biases and prejudices are not formed in isolation; they are the product of a complex dance between power and knowledge. Again, we explore this further in the next two chapters; however, for now, you can think of a dominant discourse as the story of what is labeled "normal"—what one should do and how one should do it. In the United States, there is a lingering (non-diverse) dominant societal discourse that a *man* and *woman should* get married, have children (in that order), and invest in a white picket fence. Dominant discourses are constituted by the views of the majority—not all.

Importantly, dominant discourses are neither Fact nor Truth; they certainly do not apply for everyone. When there is enough agreement by enough people to constitute a majority, something becomes "true." If we were to reduce it to an equation: "normal" = most* (within a given group). White and Epston's work simply highlights how we measure ourselves by societal discourses (e.g., White, 2007). Am I feminine enough? Am I thin enough? Am I a good mom if I go back to work after giving birth, or am I only a good mom if I stay home with my new baby? Exploring and challenging "normal" is at the heart of narrative therapy.

As you can see, "narrative" has different connotations whether you are thinking about it from a storytelling perspective of an individual as a character versus a societal discourse perspective of individuals making their way through life in communities. Thus it is not just the individual's story (i.e., narrative) that matters but it is also their relationship to society's discourses (i.e., narratives) that shape and reshape our identities and life practices. Clients' personal narratives are either aligning with, intersecting with, or contradicting the dominant discourse. When *our* narrative contradicts the *societal* narrative, we run into problems. We often blame ourselves when this happens, believing something is wrong with us. Again, White saw *this process* of falling prey to taken-for-granted knowledges as problematic. The problem is the problem. The person is the person.

APPLYING DOMINANT DISCOURSES IN CONTEXT

Consider, for instance, the following example which showcases the discourse of what a family should look like.

Person A: "A happy family is one that says, "I love you" all the time.
Person B: "That's '*a*' definition of a happy family, not '*the*' definition of a happy family."

According to social constructionism, no definition is an absolute definition. Therefore, whatever definition you have of a "happy family" is influenced by your experiences, interpretations, and your relationship to the dominant discourse. Our clients get caught up in these dominant discourses—stories of *"should's"* and *"ought to's."* In order to explore their *should's* and *ought to's*, a narrative therapist invites them to explore their values. They may ask, "Where did you learn that from?." Madigan provided some examples of questions a narrative therapist might ask a client about "what it means to be a man" (2019, p. 75):

- "What are the practices of life and ways of thinking about life that stand behind this word/term (that they have described regarding being a man)?
- Are there certain ways that you live because of this particular way of thinking?
- What are these ways of living (men's practices)?
- How do these ways of living have you relating to yourself?
- Do these ways of living bring you closer in or further away (to yourself or others)?" (p. 75)

A NON-PATHOLOGIZING STANCE: SKEPTICISM TOWARD DIAGNOSES

White emphasized the history of science and psychology as well as the effects of power and knowledge in communities. In that vein, let us examine how diagnoses are given by mental health professionals, from a narrative therapy lens. A mental health professional has gained extra knowledge to make a diagnosis; the expert knowledge on diagnoses affords them permission to make the decision to diagnose a patient as well as what to diagnose them with. This practice of power (i.e., diagnosing) perpetuates the knowledge (in this case of diagnoses and what we do with them) on a larger scale.

An obvious cautionary example is the entry of homosexuality (i.e., "ego-dystonic homosexuality") in the Diagnostic and Statistical Manual of Mental Disorders (DSM) until the late 1980s (Margolin, 2023). A mental health professional would need to gain enough psychological knowledge to be able to diagnose someone; meanwhile, their diagnosis is an exercise of power that reinforces this knowledge. Their diagnosis of sexual deviation would both operate under *and* perpetuate the knowledges-derived discourse that homosexuality is a disorder.

Keep in mind a second point of complexity. While the psychiatrist or mental health professional would have diagnosed this person with sexual deviance as both an exercise of power and knowledge, that person would also have voluntarily gone to the psychiatrist, abiding by the supposed knowledges of their society during that time. Their own self-imposed admittance to be "treated" would be an exercise of control and discipline to rid themselves of the supposed disorder.

White's avoidance of diagnosing children or adults—no small feat in our largely modernist world—was intentional. Although he often worked with people who had a diagnosis, attention-deficit hyperactivity disorder (ADHD) being a prominent example, he himself did not diagnose (White, 2007). My example of the DSM diagnosis of homosexuality is an intentionally provocative one to prove a point, but White upheld the same values regarding currently accepted diagnoses such as anxiety. By challenging dominant discourses, especially those of psychotherapeutic and psychiatric practices (White, 2011), narrative therapy works to bring forward clients' "future possibilities and life horizons" (White, 2007, p. 43). Madigan commented: "Research psychologist Svend Brinkmann (2016) wrote of 'diagnostic cultures' where DSM diagnoses, such as ADHD or depression, are becoming central to one's identity. Diagnosis-related stories become interwoven with everyday life, often in ways that foreclose on life possibilities" (Madigan, pp. 40–41). This is how White viewed diagnoses: as perpetuating psychological jargon and narratives that limited possibilities for living (White, 2007).

The argument for or against the DSM is not one I wish to enter here. Here we focus on the founders—White and Epston—and their opinions on the matter. According to White, we create space for maneuverability only when we step back and realize that the so-called knowledge, in this case from the DSM, is really a discourse. Although there are clear, tangible effects of what we consider to be knowledge, there is no Knowledge; furthermore, what counts as knowledge shifts over time. White believed that our professional knowledges were often ways of *othering* individuals as people who deviated from social norms. We live out our stories in such a way that our own experience is limited by society's discourses, and then our narratives take on a life of their own, so to speak. We create knowledges while also being subjected to them. Can we become something beyond our diagnoses? Must they become a part of who we are, dictating what we can and cannot do? What would the outcome be if we perpetuated this story? What could it be if we chose an alternative story?

RE-AUTHORING

Narratives are informed by the dominant cultural context. As we live in a society, we adopt understandings of the "totalizing discourses" (White, 1991) even if we do not agree with them. Hence these discourses affect our lives and how we carry out our daily activities—whether or not we want them to. White and Epston aimed to free clients of restrictive discourses and water the seeds, so to speak, of preferred narratives that would liberate instead of restricting their options for a preferred future (Madigan).

Re-authoring uses the client's memories or, more accurately, their stories and descriptions of their past (called *unique outcomes*, as discussed below)—to build upon preferred narratives that counter the restrictive dominant discourse. This process of re-authoring is both the theory of change and the goal in narrative therapy.

> Developing therapeutic solutions to problems, within the narrative frame, involves opening space for the authoring of alternative stories, the possibility of which have previously been marginalized by the dominant oppressive narrative which maintains the problem. According to this position, the process of therapeutic re-authoring personal narratives changes lives, problems and identities because personal narratives are constitutive of identity.
>
> *(Carr, 2001, p. 17)*

Re-authoring challenges the original client narrative of the person believing they or someone else is the problem. To re-author, a narrative therapist looks for knowledges and stories that have not yet received enough attention and have thus been obfuscated from the client's view by the domineering dominant discourse (White & Epston). The therapist then weaves the unacknowledged or less acknowledged stories—termed *subjugated stories/subjugated narratives*—together into a new story *with* the client (not *for* the client as in a reframe). Re-authoring highlights the client's exceptional knowledges and "reorients them to aspects of their experience that contradict totalizing knowledges" of dominant discourses (White, 1991, p. 29). When a therapist re-authors, they attend to the subjugated narrative/subjugated story, thereby developing an alternative story which is more useful for the client.

Re-authoring is, in part, listening to what clients are not telling you—*the absent but implicit* (Freedman, 2012). Usually, a client will come in with a story about their lives in which they are the villain or someone else is the villain. They will usually declare the problem is a person—either themselves or another. But remember, the person is not the problem; the problem is the problem. Therefore, part of re-authoring is guiding the client's ear. As reported by John Winslade and Lorraine Hedtke's workshop notes on White's last workshop:

> White is constantly on the lookout for points of entry to these subordinate stories so that they can become known, so that they can emerge from the shadows of dominant stories, so that they can become more visible.
>
> *(Winslade & Hedtke, 2008, p. 6)*

Once the subjugated stories are more visible, the client can reclaim their story, thereby no longer needing a long-term therapist. A narrative therapist does not work to *convince* the client to see the restricting dominant discourses the way the therapist sees them. They simply focus on bringing it to light for the client to reflect upon.

Narrative therapists ask questions, sometimes similar to those of a young child: "Why?." For example, you would ask, "Why did this strike you as so significant?" instead of assuming you know the reason it is significant (White, 1991, p. 38). Such questions allow the clients to hear themselves and reflect upon their own answers. As a therapist, you do not provide the perfect reframe for a client, wrapped up in a pretty bow. Rather, you respect the client's autonomy in creating their new story. The narrative therapist merely acts as a co-creator or co-author who asks about the things that are significant to the client. To re-author, you simply support your client in developing their desired narrative. The storied *events* ("historical facts," a modernist might say) stay the same, but the lines drawn to connect them can be erased and redrawn, connecting the dots in different ways. Alternative stories beget "new meanings that persons will experience as more helpful, satisfying, and open-ended" (White & Epston, p. 15).

UNIQUE OUTCOMES—NOT EXCEPTIONS

Narrative therapy's *"unique outcomes"* are different from solution focused brief therapy's (SFBT) *"exceptions."* On the one hand, unique outcomes—also called "sparkling moments" (Van Wyk, 2008)—are the descriptions that tell a counter-story to the dominant narrative. Because unique outcomes challenge the dominant discourse, they contain a more political undertone. Unique outcomes are stories that the client has not paid enough attention to because these moments have been overshadowed. The story has been subjugated. David Denborough, Co-Director of the Dulwich Centre in Australia, described how unique outcomes are used to "intensify the preferred self" (Denborough, 2019, p. 27) in creating alternative storylines. As White (2007) described, "Among other things, conversations that highlight unique outcomes provide people with the opportunity to give voice to intentions for their own lives and to develop a stronger familiarity with what they accord value to in life" (p. 220). This to key to unique outcomes.

On the other hand, exceptions in SFBT are times when the problem was not a problem or simply times when the problem was not occurring. Steve de Shazer described exceptions as "what happens when the complaint does not happen" (1986, p. 215, as cited in Korman et al., p. 5). SFBT highlights exceptions to show the client they have already done something in one context such that it proves the client can do it again in the present and future. The exception is used as encouragement to do more of what works. Therefore, we can think of unique outcomes as exceptions in our short-hand language, but that is not the complete picture.

Whereas an SFBT therapist might say, "Wow, you must be really strong to have overcome so much," a narrative therapist would be hesitant to compliment the client, being aware of the potential harm it could do. For example, there is a discourse about Black women needing to be strong, and this discourse can limit an individual's experience or gloss over the nuance of a person's lived experience and all its complexities. It can perpetuate a stifling stereotype built on oversimplification and systemic racism. Because of the narrative therapists' meticulous attention to language and discourse, the narrative therapist would instead ask, "What did that mean to you?" or "Is that a good thing or a bad thing?" Keeping the focus on the client, the narrative therapist does not assume the meaning of an experience for a client. In no way would the narrative therapist attempt to convince the client of the therapist's perspective or to realize how great things are if they only looked at it from a different point of view. Narrative therapists listen for unique outcomes as the dots they are trying to connect. Re-authoring unique outcomes allows the client the opportunity to recreate a new relationship with the problem, not just do something differently.

LANDSCAPE OF ACTION AND LANDSCAPE
OF CONSCIOUSNESS/IDENTITY

Landscape of action and **landscape of consciousness** are two narrative terms of literary derivation that are often confused but need not be.

> Landscape of action questions encourage persons to situate unique outcomes in sequences of events that unfold across time according to particular plots. Landscape of consciousness questions encourage persons to reflect on and to determine the meaning of those developments that occur in the landscape of action.
>
> *(White, 1991, p. 30)*

Oversimplifying for my new learners: landscape of action is the action—plot—and landscape of consciousness is the meaning (1991). Getting into a bit more depth, White's landscape of action comes from Bruner's ideas about how humans are story-telling beings that story (as a verb) sequences of events across time (White, 2005). The *fabula* connects the events.

> In any case of the fabula of a story—its timeless underlying theme—seems to be a unity that incorporates at least three constituents. It contains a plight into which characters have fallen as a result of intentions that have gone awry either because of circumstances, of the "character of characters," or most likely of the interaction between the two. What gives the story its unity is the manner in which plight, characters, and consciousness interact to yield a structure that has a start, development, and a "sense of ending."
>
> *(White, 2007, p. 21, as cited in Duvall & Berés, p. 52)*

The landscape of consciousness is composed of meaning and identity conclusions, connected through the fabula, creating a narrative. Clients treat these narratives as True.

Narrative therapists try to elicit as much detail as possible. These rich story descriptions are called *thick descriptions*. Thick descriptions, as opposed to thin descriptions (see Geertz), are full of meanings: purpose, hopes, values, beliefs, and desires. Thick descriptions are desirable so that "people's lives are thickened and more deeply rooted in history, the gaps are filled, and the storylines are clearly named" (White, 2005, p. 10). This is also the thread that connects unique outcomes—the sparkling moments.

When you re-author, you thicken the alternative story—the preferred narrative—using unique comes (Marsten et al., 2016). A quick note: according to a modernist, the landscape of action are the Facts of the person's life. According to a social constructionist who sees everything as storied, there are no such things; everything is interpretative. Carr included some examples of questions a narrative therapist may ask to thicken descriptions:

1. Can you tell me your memory of that? (landscape of action)
2. What was happening before this event and what happened afterward? (landscape of action)
3. At what point in your life did this occur? (landscape of action)
4. If your problem was a project, what would you call it? (landscape of action)
5. What does this story say about you as a person? (landscape of consciousness)

6. What does this story say about your relationship with your mother/father/sibling? (landscape of consciousness)
7. How did that effect you? (landscape of consciousness)
8. Was that a good thing for your relationship or a bad thing? (landscape of consciousness) (pp. 26–27)

RE-MEMBERING, DEFINITIONAL CEREMONY, AND OUTSIDER WITNESS PRACTICE

Re-membering has anthropological roots (see Myerhoff; White, 2005) and refers to the club or group to which one belongs. Narrative therapy involves reviewing one's memberships and often is about re-engaging with a significant person (2005). Who was the significant person to the client? What tracks and impressions did they leave on the client's life? Cultivating a thick description helps a narrative therapist be able to have others in the story who contribute to the client's preferred narrative, regardless of whether they are physically in the room or even alive.

Definitional ceremonies refer back to public celebrations of therapeutic achievements. It is a means by which clients can show "themselves" by telling their new story. Alternatively, they may sit back and hear their story through the ears of another. When a group of people listen to the client and state (not complimentarily but authentically) what they have heard, they are participating in a new story construction about who that person is. This is narrative therapy's *outsider witness* practice. As the descriptions are thickened, so are preferred identity conclusions.

One can hear the similarities to Andersen's reflecting team practices in White's (2007) description: "Outsider witnesses engage one another in conversations about the expressions of the telling they were drawn to, about the images that these expressions evoked, about the personal experiences that resonated with these expressions" (p. 165). White's purpose in arranging outsider witness retellings was to have clients self-affirm in their retelling of their story rather than have the therapist affirm the client is "good," "doing well," or "on the right track." Those latter options would mistakenly have the narrative therapist playing out a modernist therapist's role as an expert that is, employing an expert stance.

DECONSTRUCTION

Deconstruction originated from a philosopher and linguist named Jacques Derrida (pronounced "deh-ree-dah"). As a linguist, Derrida used the method of deconstruction to examine how words work in texts, and deconstruction involved a thorough, complex analysis. It challenges assumptions we often have about how words work, especially our tendency to think of words' meaning as fixed. Derrida's work showed how binaries or seeming opposites ("light" and "dark") are interrelated and interdependent.

White's version of deconstruction does not align with Derrida's model of analysis (White, 1991); however, White still used it as a helpful term to describe part of what he was doing in therapy. He said:

> According to my rather loose definition, deconstruction has to do with procedures that subvert taken-for-granted realities and practices; those so-called "truths"

that are split off from the conditions and the context of their production, those disembodied ways of speaking that hide their biases and prejudices, and those familiar practices of self and of relationship that are subjugating of persons' lives.

(1991, p. 27)

White's version of deconstruction in narrative therapy explores how dominant discourses have got a hold on a client's life. In this type of deconstruction, the dominant narrative is investigated, perhaps subtly challenged through curious questions and connections. The problem-saturated story (Carr) is processed and broken down through careful analysis of its assumptions. The problem itself is externalized as something outside the individual, and together new narratives are co-created (i.e., co-authored). The problem, not the person, is objectified and personified (Marsten et al., 2016). We delve into deconstruction and externalization in Chapter 6.

EXTERNALIZATION

Separating the person from the problem is *externalization* and the narrative therapy conversations in which the problem, not the person, is objectified are called *externalizing conversations*. Through externalization, clients are challenged to pull from their own knowledges—experiences within their cultures, sub-cultures, and personal stories that may counter the dominant discourse. A narrative therapist might ask, "What does this success in resisting the influence of the problem tell us about you as a person?" (Carr, p. 25). This helps them see the influence of the problem on their lives and see how the problem has shaped their view of themselves and others.

By separating their identity from the objectifying dominant narrative(s) that tells them they are flawed, clients have more freedom to create and move within alternative, empowering narratives. When therapists externalize the problem, they can join forces with the client to, for example, "tame the problem," "reeducate the problem," "resign from the problem's service," "reduce the problem's grip on their lives," and so on (White, 2007, p. 33). In general, one should avoid a battle metaphor (p. 32) because it sets one up against oneself.

A THOUGHT EXPERIMENT

When Alice Morgan was learning to practice narrative therapy, she had to practice thinking in a different way. She explained it as follows:

> I visualized "the Worry," or "the Depression," or "the Bickering" as a separate and distinct image and this allowed me to change my language and begin to more easily ask externalizing questions. Feeling this distance between the person and the problem allowed me space to practice new ways of speaking.
>
> *(Morgan, p. 88)*

Now, let us examine another example, this time from Epston's work. Here is Epston's example of externalization during an interview (i.e., session) with a young girl and her mother:

> Well, here's my thinking. I have to assume that the problem, whatever it might be, is no pushover. And we might have to join together if we are going to do

anything about it. But before we can even think about teaming up, it would be good for me to know what Francine's "wonderfulnesses" are, so we can all see what she has going for her and consider how to put that against the problem.

(Martsen et al., p. 36)

Similarly, White emphasized a respectful understanding of the problem as separate from the person. Building on this, let us consider a thought experiment where Michael White is your supervisor.

A young woman comes and explains her presenting problems: "I am anorexic and have been for the past four years, and now that I've graduated college and moved back in with my family, I'm anxious *all* the time." White would likely caution you to not to consider this client "anorexic" and "anxious." Instead, he would encourage you to think about her as someone who has historically had problems related to eating who is experiencing something that she has chosen to call anxiety. By shifting how the therapist thinks about the client in this manner, White would be encouraging you to practice anti-objectification of her and thus not to think of her as the problem. White would instead "map the effects of the problem" and ask questions about how "The Anorexia" and "The Anxiety" have played a role in her life. He might nudge you to ask about how Anorexia has taken up so much space in her life and in what ways Anorexia's presence has gotten in the way of some things she wanted to do. Regarding the anxiety, you might consider asking something along the lines of, "What has your Anxiety been convincing you is the truth about yourself and your circumstances?" Can you see how this is externalizing the problem *outside of her* rather than conceptualizing her as being the problem (which would be internalizing the problem)? Speaking like this, you have already begun *externalizing conversations*.

As your supervisor, White might ask you what you think may be some of the effects of her internalization of the problem. After thinking it over, you might say how seeing herself as the problem might strengthen a relationship to shame and make her feel like "a failure" for "not trying hard enough," "not being strong enough," or "never following through." Here is where deconstruction becomes clear. As a new therapist under White's wing, you begin to understand how those quotes that came to your mind are societal narratives—discourses that may be limiting the client's possibilities for a richer story such that she may see herself as *lazy*, *weak*, or *a quitter*. Additionally, as you continue your conversation with her, you start to piece together that her poor relationship with eating may relate to the dominant discourse (which is ever-evolving over time) that women should be thin to be attractive (which is merely one of the dominant discourses). You realize that part of her current story is that she "needs to be" "attractive," and to become attractive, according to the discourse, she "has to be" "thin." Ideally, you understand how she has her own complex web of experiences, but you see how this discourse has left an imprint on her.

Part of your narrative therapist stirring would be to deconstruct this narrative and get her to see whether she wants this narrative in her life and to what extent. A simple question like, "Where did you first learn that in order to be attractive one has to be thin?" can open up huge possibilities to *deconstruct* what is "truth" and where this "truth" came from, moving toward what is true *for her*. Where you go next, constructing her journey with her, is *re-authoring*. You will collaborate with her through co-authoring a new narrative that opens space for stories about who she is. This is no longer an anorexic, anxious woman. This is Analise, who loves dogs, hiking, and architecture and who, through your narrative conversations, realizes she does not need to date a "man" (a discourse), be married by 25 (a discourse), and/or be "thin" (a discourse) for someone to date, love, and marry her (a discourse). Remember, discourses leave us with *"should's."* The exact narrative does not matter so long as it remains *her* narrative, a more helpful story that counters the dominant discourse. As a narrative therapist, you act as a co-author, listening out for things that were already in her story but were not emphasized because the dominant discourses were taking up all the room. You guide her in creating a more empowering story where she has a different understanding of and relationship to the problem than it being *her.*

SUMMARY

An essential component of narrative therapy is to avoid dehumanization. Technically speaking, you aim to avoid the "objectification of people" (as problems). The narrative therapist identifies the problem the client has *internalized* and deconstructs the dominant discourses that *objectify* people (i.e., as objects). Narrative therapists are incredibly attuned to language and endlessly curious about the meaning that clients make of their experiences. Part of the responsibility of a narrative therapist is intentionality (Duvall & Béres, 2011): to maintain constant awareness of the language one uses to avoid harm to clients. Accidental or not, reinforcing limiting dominant discourses can have devastating effects on clients.

Narrative therapy involves externalizing the problem as the problem, deconstructing the dominant discourse(s), identifying and exploring unique outcomes, and thickening the subjugated story to build upon an alternative, preferred narrative. Narrative therapists work to collaboratively re-author narratives with clients, providing them opportunity for stories that embolden self-agency. The specific new narrative is not as important as "a" new and useful narrative. If you are interested in a deeper explanation of narrative therapy in practice, I encourage you to read Michael White's and David Epston's primary sources and works by the renowned authors at the end of this chapter such as Jill Freedman, Gene Combs, Stephen Madigan, Alice Morgan, and David Denborough.

REFLECTIVE QUESTIONS

1. Narrative therapy introduced the language of a decentered yet influential position; meanwhile, C-DP introduced the not-knowing stance. Compare and contrast these. How might they converge in narrative therapy?
2. What opportunities does the decentered, influential position provide for the therapist and client?
3. In narrative therapy, the person is not the problem. How does this complement a non-pathologizing stance?
4. How does a narrative therapist help clients reclaim their lives?
5. How do you choose what to re-author?

Keywords

Decentered

Influential

Discourse/Narrative/Story

Dominant Discourse/Dominant Narrative/Dominant Story

Subjugated Discourse/Subjugated Story

Unique Outcomes

Landscape of Action

Landscape of Consciousness

Re-Authoring

Deconstruction

Externalization

Narrative Therapy Post-Test (Inspired by Madigan & Epston, 1995)

1. Whose expertise is valued in narrative therapy?
   a. A narrative therapist privileges the client's expertise on their own life. This is called adopting a non-expert stance. C-DP also adopts a non-expert stance.
2. How does narrative therapy think change is possible?
   a. Narrative therapists believe nothing is static and change occurs through stories, linking events across time.
3. How does narrative therapy deal with contradictions?
   a. Narrative therapy is multi-voiced and "multi-storied" (White, 2007). Contradictions do not necessarily require attention unless they are in relation to a dominant discourse that needs to be deconstructed.
4. How do I know which alternative story to build upon?
   a. Narrative therapy is done collaboratively, leading from behind. There is no one story to re-author. There are many paths to re-authoring a client's story, and many points of entry.
5. In what ways can hermeneutic processes be involved?
   a. Like, C-DP, narrative therapists engage in reflexive work where the interpretation of past, present, and future are always a part of therapy, influencing the therapeutic process moment-by-moment.
6. What responsibility does the therapist have?
   a. The narrative therapist has a responsibility to not perpetuate limiting dominant discourses that narrow clients' outcomes. Narrative therapists must have a heightened awareness about the language they use. The therapist is not tied to a specific outcome in a behavioral sense but is concerned with building upon the subjugated story and cultivating clients' self-agency.
7. How much direction does the narrative therapist provide on the client's alternative story?
   a. A narrative therapist re-authors *with* the client, not *for* the client. They primarily do so by asking meaningful questions instead of making statements, offering advice/directives, or initiating therapeutic interventions. White and Epston were preoccupied with avoiding infringing upon a client's autonomy.

8. How does a narrative therapist get a client to see deeper into themselves or have a deeper understanding of who they are?

   a. This is a misunderstanding of narrative therapy. They do not attempt to change a client's so-called internal identity but rather believe in multi-storied individuals with the capacity for many identities. Importantly, narrative therapists do not believe an identity, nor personality for that matter, lies within a person. Narrative therapy holds a relational view of identity construction (and reconstruction) in communities. There is no "deeper," only different—and hopefully more helpful.

9. Does a narrative therapist just ask, "And then what happened?"

   a. No, narrative therapists want to know what happened, how it happened, and why it happened. Importantly, the answers to these questions should be filled in by the client(s), not therapist. The emphasis is on the client's meaning-making. As clients speak on their experiences, they reflect on them, and "the act of reflecting on the events and experiences of life is the landscape of consciousness" (Duvall & Berés, p. 50).

MICHAEL WHITE AND DAVID EPSTON: PRIMARY SOURCES

Epston, D., Carlson, T. S., & polanco, m. (2019). Re-imagining narrative therapy: An ecology of magic and mystery for the maverick. *Journal of Narrative Family Therapy, 3,* 1–18.

Freeman, J., Epston, D., & Lobovits, D. (1997). *Playful approaches to serious problems.* W. W. Norton.

Madigan, S., & Epston, D. (1995). From spy-chiatric gaze to communities of concern: From professional monologue to dialogue. In S. Friedman (Ed.), *The reflecting team in action: Collaborative practice in family therapy* (pp. 257–276). Guilford Press.

Marsten, D., Epston, D., & Markham, L. (2016). *Narrative therapy in Wonderland: Connecting with children's imaginative know-how.* W. W. Norton.

White, M. (1991). Deconstruction and therapy. *Dulwich Centre Newsletter, 3,* 21–40.

White, M. (2005). *Workshop notes.* www.dulwichcentre.com.au

White, M. (2007). *Maps of narrative practice.* W. W. Norton.

White, M. (2011). *Narrative practice: Continuing the conversations* (dig. ed.). W. W. Norton & Company.

White, M. (2012). Scaffolding a therapeutic conversation. In T. Malinen, S. J. Cooper, & F. N. Thomas (Eds.), *Masters of narrative and collaborative therapies: The voices of Andersen, Anderson, and White* (dig. ed., pp. 113–150). Routledge.

White, M., & Epston, D. (1990). *Narrative means to therapeutic ends.* W. W. Norton.

White, M., & Morgan, A. (2006). *Narrative therapy with children and their families.* Dulwich Centre Publications.

Renowned Sources

Anderson, H. (2015). Postmodern/poststructural/social construction therapies: Collaborative, narrative, and solution-focused. In T. L. Sexton & J. Lebow (Ed.), *Handbook of family therapy: The science and practice of working with families and couples* (1st dig. ed., pp. 182–204). Routledge

Carr, A. (2001). *Michael White's narrative therapy.* Edwin Mellen Press.

Combs, G., & Freedman, J. (1996). *Narrative therapy: The social construction of preferred realities.* W. W. Norton.

Combs, G., & Freedman, J. (2012). Narrative, poststructuralism, and social justice: Current practices in narrative therapy. *The Counseling Psychologist, 40*(7), 1033–1060.

Denborough, D. (2019). Travelling down the neuro-pathway: Narrative practice, neuroscience, bodies, emotions, and the affective turn. *The International Journal of Narrative Therapy and Community Work, 3*, 1–120. https://dulwichcentre.com.au/wp-content/uploads/2022/05/International-Journal-of-Narrative-Therapy-2019-Issue3.pdf

Duvall, J., & Béres, L. (2011). *Innovations in narrative therapy: Connecting practice, training, and research* (dig. ed.). W. W. Norton & Company.

Freedman, J. (2012). Explorations of the absent but implicit. *International Journal of Narrative Therapy & Community Work, 4*, 1–10.

Haley, J. (2010). *Uncommon therapy: The psychiatric techniques of Milton Erickson.* W. W. Norton.

Hibel, J., & polanco, m. (2010). Tuning the ear: Listening in narrative therapy. *Journal of Systemic Therapies, 29*(1), 51–66.

Korman, H., De Jong, P., & Jordan, S. S. (2020). Steve de Shazer's theory development. *Journal of Solution Focused Practices, 4*(2), 47–70.

Madigan, S. (2019). *Narrative therapy* (2nd dig. ed.). American Psychological Association.

Malinen, T., Cooper, S. J., & Thomas, F. N. (Eds.). (2012). *Masters of narrative and collaborative therapies: The voices of Andersen, Anderson, and White* (dig. ed.). Routledge.

Morgan, A. (2002). Beginning to use a narrative approach in therapy. *International Journal of Narrative Therapy and Community Work, 1*, 85–90.

Winslade, J., & Hedtke, L. (2008). Michael White: Fragments of an event, *The International Journal of Narrative Therapy and Community Work, 2*, 5–11, https://dulwichcentre.com.au/product/michael-white-fragments-of-an-event-john-winslade-lorraine-hedtke-with-an-introduction-by-david-epston/

Additional References

Boston, P. (2018). Systemic family therapy and the influence of post-modernism. *Advances in Psychiatric Treatment, 6*(6), 450–457.

Dowling, E., & Vetere, A. (2016). Narrative concepts and therapeutic challenges. In A. Vetere & E. Dowling (Eds.), *Narrative therapies with children and their families: A practitioner's guide to concepts and approaches* (2nd dig. ed., pp. 3–27). Routledge.

Ilic, D. (2017). *Conversation analysis of Michael White's decentered and influential position.* Nova Southeastern University. https://nsuworks.nova.edu/shss_dft_etd/25.

Margolin, L. (2023). The third backdoor: How the *DSM casebooks* pathologized homosexuality. *Journal of Homosexuality, 70*(2), 291–306.

Pare, D. (2012). *The practice of collaborative counseling and psychotherapy: Developing skills in culturally mindful helping.* Sage.

Rustin, M., & Rustin, M. (2016). In A. Vetere & E. Dowling (Eds.). (2016). *Narrative therapies with children and their families: A practitioner's guide to concepts and approaches* (2nd dig. ed., pp. 3–27). Routledge.

Van Wyk, R. (2008). Narrative house: A metaphor for narrative therapy. A tribute to Michael White. https://repository.up.ac.za/bitstream/handle/2263/8828/VanWyk_Narrative%282008%29.pdf?sequence=1

Vetere, A., & Dowling, E. (Eds.). (2016). *Narrative therapies with children and their families: A practitioner's guide to concepts and approaches* (2nd dig. ed.). Routledge.

Wand, G., & Pepe, T. (2023). An introductory guide to skillful therapist positioning. *Journal of Systemic Therapies, 42*(1), 18–37.

CHAPTER 5

Michel Foucault

....

Remember, as you read through these chapters, you can always return to the Introduction to refresh your memory on the terms you learned such as epistemology and social constructionism.

QUESTIONS TO THINK ABOUT

1. What are the primary texts associated with Foucault?
2. In what ways was Foucault provocative for his time? And today?
3. What is the relationship between power and knowledge as Foucault sees it?
4. What is the relationship between discourse and control?
5. What are "docile bodies?"

Michel Foucault (phonetically pronounced "mee-shell foo-kow") was a famous French thinker—an academic, philosopher, historian, and social theorist whose works had major societal impacts. Foucault's ideas blur the boundaries between historical analysis, social commentary, and political activism. In this section, I deferred primarily to the biographical information shared by David Macey (2019), whose outstanding biography was written with the collaboration of Foucault's former lover and long-term partner and is seen as a true-to-life account. I also incorporated authors who are known, reputable sources who have written extensively on Foucault: Gary Gutting (2019), Stuart Elden (2021, 2023), Eric Paras (2020), Paul Oliver (2010), and Robert Hurley (2020). Finally, I have included tertiary support from supplemental, modern-day resources.

Because of Foucault's long list of written and transcribed works, there are many ideas one could underscore as critical to understanding Foucault. There is an additional complication that Foucault himself changed over time, no doubt indicated by the title of Macey's biography: *The Lives of Michel Foucault*. Therefore, my explanation will

DOI: 10.4324/9781003439349-8

surely fall short of encompassing all of Foucault's ideas. Thus this chapter outlines the concepts I believe are the most central to Michael White's interpretation of Foucauldian thought and are the most relevant to modern-day postmodern family therapists.

WHO WAS MICHEL FOUCAULT?

Michel Foucault was born in provincial France in 1929. Foucault had a privileged upbringing with an esteemed family where his father's position as a well-respected physician afforded young Foucault more rigorous academic opportunities than would otherwise be available, allowing Foucault entry into the prestigious Sorbonne as well as affording him opportunities for world travel at a young age (Gutting). Nevertheless, Foucault had a complicated relationship with his bourgeois roots. Being both the son of a revered surgeon and the grandson of a surgeon/anatomy professor (Elden, 2021), one might have assumed Foucault would enter the medical profession himself. However, much to the chagrin of his father, Foucault denied this route in favor of the humanities and his brother Denys, five years his junior, became a surgeon instead (Macey). Depending on the commentator, Foucault had either distaste or disdain for his authoritarian father, from whom he certainly craved distance and disassociation, regardless of the opportunities his father's social position brought him. Illustratively, from a young age Foucault refused to take on the tradition of the firstborn sons' adoption of the name "Paul" and would insist on being called "Michel" throughout his life (Macey).

Foucault was a competitive student who excelled in history, French, German, English, Latin, Greek, and philosophy (Elden, 2021), but not without cost. Since he was a young schoolboy, Foucault had nightmares that he could not perform well academically, as measured by his inability to read the text in front of him (Macey). His recurring dream shows the intensity with which Foucault approached academia as well as recognition as an intellectual. Unsurprisingly, Foucault advanced in academic spheres, becoming a professor of and eventually chair of philosophy, where he gave himself the title: "Professor of the History of Systems of Thought" (Paras, p. 3).

Although in the end it was not his chosen career choice to become a psychologist, Foucault earned degrees in psychology as well as philosophy, and he still dabbled in considerations of becoming a psychologist or psychiatrist even into the 1950s. According to Macey, at one point, he held an unofficial internship position at a clinical mental hospital, and at another point, he used his connections to work in a prison where he analyzed psychological exams to review for risks of suicidality and determine whether "specialist units" were called for. While working at the former, he developed a friendship with a patient named Roger, who was lobotomized after drugs had no effect on his depressive state and which "left Foucault with an indelible image of suffering and which, given Foucault's own depressive tendencies, must have had a considerable impact and left the would-be psychiatrist wondering whether death might not be preferable to Roger's non-existence" (pp. 80–81). Meanwhile, at the latter site, Foucault assisted psychiatrist Jacqueline Verdeaux, sometimes donning a lab coat, and contributing to data comprising inmates' psychological profiles, sometimes assisting with neurological exams "to try to distinguish between real and simulated psychopathological, and particularly epileptic, disorders" (pp. 81–82). His experiences at the hospital and prison in the 1950s unquestionably had lasting effects. Working at those internships affected the way Foucault thought about institutions and the knowledge perpetuated by them.

As Elden (2021) informed his readers, ten years after Foucault entered academia and had become an instructor, Foucault finally published his labor of love: his university thesis *Folie et dèraison: Histoire de la folie à l'âge Classique* aka *Madness and Civilization: A History of Insanity in the Age of Reason*. This book highlighted his cross-sectional interests in history, philosophy, psychology, and literature. *Madness and Civilization* would also be the turning point which heralded Foucault as a counter-culture figure (Elden, 2023; Gutting; Sabot, 2023).

In 1981, Foucault openly discussed his lifelong attraction to men and his "worry-desire" about it (Macey, p. 37), which certainly makes sense given the controversy surrounding gay relationships in the 1940s when Foucault came into adulthood up until the mid-1980s when Foucault died. He passed only a couple of years after homosexuality had been taken out of the DSM.

According to many commentators such as Nabulsi (2019), Foucault was also interested in bondage, domination, and sadomasochism (BDSM). Although Foucault's first "friend" was in Paris in 1946, since he lived in a time when this was heavily stigmatized and pathologized in France and elsewhere in the Western world, Foucault was discreet about his sexual affairs with men until his late life (Macey).

When one reads Foucault's biographies, it is not much of a leap to assume Foucault's personal experiences of being on both sides of mental health care in his 20s influenced his interest in the history and practices of psychology and psychiatry. Indeed, most of those familiar with Foucault's life or works draw this conclusion. If any additional evidence were needed, Foucault himself said, "My books have always been my personal problems with madness, with prisons, and with sexuality" (as cited in Macey, p. 11).

WHAT DID FOUCAULT WRITE?

Foucault's seminal work is *Madness and Civilization* (1961). It is still one of his most famous books, along with *The Birth of the Clinic* (1963), *Discipline and Punish* (1975), and his multi-volume series titled *The History of Sexuality* (1976+). Although you can certainly find Foucault's ideas in other places such as lectures and compiled notes, these books are among his most cited and most celebrated (Hurley, 2020).

WHAT ARE THE PROMINENT FOUCAULDIAN CONCEPTS?

Knowledge

Foucault's affinity for history is well documented. Foucault, often viewed as a historian in his own right, was particularly interested in the history of knowledge: the transformation of knowledge over time. Foucault had an unconventional view on knowledge. The *knowledge* Foucault spoke about is not what we might term True or empirical. Crossing over with social constructionism, he believed that whatever was the knowledge of the time would be replaced by different knowledge across time. Rather than considering knowledge to be the summation of facts, transferred from one person to another person or group of people, Foucault saw knowledge like history: a particular story or set of stories within a particular society which were enacted in a particular point in time.

History, he maintained, is constructed communally. To me, it brings to mind the phrase, "History is written by the victors." It could never be the case that we have an objective history because what we call history is a collection of stories told from an individual's or group's perspective. And even an individual's telling of history would not negate that the individual belongs to a larger group which shapes how they experience the events. Although this was clearly outlined by even the very first known historian, Herodotus, many forget that history is open to interpretation. *Discourses* are not *facts*, and this idea resonated with White. We discuss discourses more in this chapter.

To understand Foucault, we must see the parallel between history and knowledge. Neither history nor knowledge is a collection of facts; furthermore, neither history nor knowledge is rational. To try to capture where Foucault was going with this, perhaps we could revise the aforementioned phrase ("History is written by the victors") to become: "*Knowledge* is dictated by the victors/dominant group." Knowledge does not exist in isolation; it is a malleable social process that is a product of its time. For this reason, Foucault called himself an "archeologist" of knowledge. He was interested in the excavation, so to speak, of the knowledges of a time. He exhumed "particular ways of acting or thinking that presuppose a specific pattern of knowledge, which then becomes characteristic of a particular historical period" (Oliver, pp. 26–27). Foucault did not believe in Knowledge (capital "K") but in knowledges (lowercase "k"; pluralized) at particular times. This is critical to understanding narrative therapy.

Knowledges change when nonconformists, the outliers, gain enough of a following to become the predominant group. Although labels are anathema to Foucault and—as a client once told me, "We would not want to ruffle the feathers of Foucault!"—this is, or at least fits with, social constructionism. He might never have called himself a social constructionist; however, many of his ideas align with social constructionist ideas, including a detestation for classification where a label comes to be accepted for "what it is."

Discourse

Foucault was heavily interested in epistemology and the *processes* by which knowledge is created and maintained. What we consider Knowledge, he argued, is shaped by *discourse*. And discourses are passed down by institutions that reinforce certain understandings and activities. The predominant discourses determine and are determined by social norms.

Here is an example to refresh your memory. Elementary schools in the United States use textbooks to teach certain subjects. Both the books chosen and what is taught are determined by greater authorities. We immediately think of the teachers who run the classes, but then there are the principals who run the school and then the larger school board. Even the government is involved in what is taught in schools and how. Curriculum, textbooks, and teaching methods all reinforce certain discourses, which students understand to be Knowledge, which students are then tested on to make sure they understand said "knowledge." Foucault called for us to analyze the institutions— schools, universities, prisons, psychiatric institutions, and the government—that were determining what was acceptable knowledge and shaping how we view the world.

Notably, his purpose was to point them out for individuals to make up their own minds, not dictate new Knowledge.

Foucault's use of discourse refers to the social stories that affect how we live our lives. The predominant discourse is often seen as Knowledge; making it so knowledge and discourse are inherently in a relationship with power. Knowledge and discourse are intertwined themselves and further intertwined with power.

Power

Michel Foucault wrote extensively about his coined term "pouvoir-savoir" or *"power-knowledge"* (aka "knowledge-power"). His conceptualization resonated with people across disciplines such as sociology, psychology, political science, and philosophy. Rather than seeing these two as completely unrelated, Foucault believed knowledge and power engage in a recursive dance: "The exercise of power perpetually creates knowledge and, conversely, knowledge constantly induces effects of power" (Foucault, 1980, p. 52). Foucault said, "It is impossible for knowledge not to engender power" (p. 52).

From a Foucauldian standpoint, power and knowledge are not individual nouns. They are mutually reinforcing activities. Institutions determine knowledge by creating and perpetuating the prevailing or dominant discourses of the time. And the dominant discourses shape our power structures by determining who is perceived as a legitimate authority to establish and maintain social norms. The power structures will control what is disseminated as knowledge. And institutions will necessarily marginalize and often silence the voices of outliers who do not fall under the dominant discourse's idea of what is socially acceptable—as determined by "knowledge."

Neither knowledge nor power can be inert. It would be impossible for them to be stagnant or stationary in any way due to their constant cyclical nature. Recall our conversation in the first chapter on recursivity as it aligned with Harlene Anderson's, Tom Andersen's, and Lynn Hoffman's ideas related to reflexive *withness* practices. Although it would perhaps be more correct to conceptualize Foucault's cycle as mutually constitutive, it certainly bears a resemblance to the hermeneutic cycle. The difference I would point out is that while hermeneutics is interested in interpretation and the interpretation of interpretation, Foucault was interested in the action or exercises of power-knowledge. Still, his conceptualization remains similar in that knowledge and power are in a dynamic, mutually influential relationship.

If *the exercise of power* that is *executed by people in a position of power* and also *performed* in our daily activities *can change,* what we think qualifies as *knowledge would change* as the reigning power changes over time along with the activities of the masses who live in accordance with this. A simplified (although technically incorrect because it is reductive) explanation is that (1) whoever is in power changes, so (2) the rules change, and (3) what counts as knowledge will also change. Furthermore, (4) as knowledge changes, it will change the people's practices of living and behaving, and then (5) people in positions of power will be affected by this change. Now if you begin to understand this, you can alter the linear explanation above to see it as circular, just like you practiced in Chapter 1.

As Oliver put it, "Power requires knowledge to be effective, and knowledge, at the same time, generates power" (p. 42). They do not happen one at a time. They constantly, recursively, fall back on one another. This is often complicated for new learners, but this point is critical to understanding Foucault, White, and narrative therapy.

As White (2012) explained, people often mistakenly interpret Foucault as saying that knowledge *is* power, but it is not as straightforward as that. Philosophers rarely are a straightforward bunch. Foucault discussed power and knowledge as intimately interwoven as activities—with palpable societal consequences.

Understanding the power-knowledge relationship from a Foucauldian lens necessitates an understanding that it is not only the people in power that enforce power upon the people. The people are controlled, certainly, in power structures, but they also control themselves, coloring inside the lines to stay "normal," if you will, according to what the discourses are.

This gives discourses an interesting relationship with control. Societal discourses involve control because they tell us where and how we should conform; moreover, for the most part, we end up monitoring ourselves for conformity to the reigning discourses of the time. Discourses are thrust upon us at the same time we act upon them. The discourses end up controlling us because we believe them and control ourselves to conform with the discourses. And we are apt to call these forms "self-control" and "discipline." The complex social dynamics in play in Western societies have created, as Foucault termed it, *"docile bodies"* who are controlled, in a sense, by their own self-monitoring/adherence to the reigning discourses they are operating under; meanwhile, their practices perpetuate this power-knowledge (aka knowledge-power) relationship (Foucault, 1995).

One can conceptualize discourses as the reigning knowledges of a particular society at a particular time. Thinking about societal knowledges as social discourses helps emphasize the difference between static Knowledge and malleable knowledges.

CAUTIONARY COMMENTARY

I caution my readers against common takeaways from Foucault which are often misaligned from what I believe he meant. By using knowledge-power, Foucault was referring to the relationship of two separate things interacting together that become something different when they interact (Foucault, 1980). Neither did Foucault see power as something someone had internally within themselves or within a position. He saw *practices* of power—on all members' parts—perpetuating discourses. There is also a misconception that the reason Foucault brought people's attention to power structures in society was to support revolts or encourage a challenge to the powerful figures at the top. That was neither Foucault's conceptualization nor purpose—although Foucault was praised as an activist, and Foucault's ideas have influenced the development of post-structuralism and feminist movements and conversations about power in society. He did not want to topple the people at the top because he knew that they would just be replaced by different other people at the top. Instead, he wanted people to think critically and be "informed consumers" about their beliefs, values, and decisions and for them to be aware of who is telling them what and why they might do so. His profound analyses of knowledge, power, discourses, and complex social interchanges led him to be a main figurehead of post-structuralism; although, like the words "gay," "activist," or seemingly any other label, Foucault never adopted that label for himself. Foucault focused on ideas instead of categories.

Finally, it is worth noting the argument that Foucault's beliefs in the real effects of power-knowledge of power might make his philosophy a dash more modern than social constructionism, even though both post-structuralism and social constructionism are undeniably postmodern for their skepticism toward grand narratives and totalizing truths. Postmodern feminism has the same critique, but that is for a different book.

BRIEF SUMMARIES AND ANALYSES OF FOUCAULT'S FAMOUS WORKS

Madness and civilization: a history of insanity in the age of reason (1961)

Foucault opened this book by exploring the history of leprosy. He discussed how those with leprosy had been quarantined from the rest of society in lazar houses, keeping the masses safe from contagion. Lepers were viewed with fear and disgust and as some-*thing* that needed to be controlled and secluded away from the rest of society.

When leprosy was eradicated, society continued the processes that were already in place: "Leprosy disappeared, the leper vanished, or almost, from memory; these structures [of what we do with people who are 'othered'] remained" (Foucault, 1988, p. 7). In the mid-1600s, madness took the place of leprosy. Madness came to be seen as a threat and became something from which to protect others. Protecting society from a physical disease evolved to protecting society from spiritual or mental dis-ease. During this period, those labeled poor or mad were seen as moral failures, neither of them allegedly contributing to society. People's lives became policed in a determination of decency and decorum.

> [Bar patrons and transient individuals] must be punished according to law and placed in houses of correction; as for those with wives and children, investigation must be made as to whether they were married and their children baptized, "for these people live like savages without being married, nor buried, nor baptized."
>
> *(as cited in Foucault, 1988, p. 50)*

Madness came to be used to describe those who would challenge convention, and society's solution toward madness was(/is) shame and seclusion.

Foucault believed that what madness "is" is not one stable thing. Madness is set within a particular society's context. We label people as "mad," "delirious," and "unreasonable" when they do not follow our societal rules. It is a judgment based upon supposed knowledge in which citizens become willing participants in maintaining the system. Who is labeled "mad" does not depend as much on the individual so much as on the discourses of the zeitgeist.

Foucault criticized punishments, especially where supposedly "unreasonable" people were sent away, and he described how un-reason itself is just a different way of rule-following, adhering to different rules. He applied the same logic to "delirium," a popular word of the era, employing its etymology to define it as deviating from the rules or expected path. He challenged the idea that unconventional people are inherently dangerous. Foucault saw a larger picture in which *what* was seen as a threat was a snapshot of the knowledges of the time.

Foucault encouraged his readers to reflect on the power behind the languaged discourses that would pervade society. Here again is the postmodern focus on language. Foucault considered society's dominant discourses as expressions of power that people simultaneously participate in while also allowing themselves to be dominated by these narratives. You can see from the quote above there was a popular religious discourse that affected society's determination of madness versus normalcy. There were severe consequences and punishments for those who deviated from the discourses of the time—just like today.

It will come as no surprise that Foucault denounced the *"medical gaze"* through which psychiatric patients are "cured." He rather vehemently challenged psychological practices, becoming strongly associated with the anti-psychiatry movement. He said, "You know the difference between a real science and pseudoscience? A real science recognizes and accepts its own history without feeling attacked. When you tell a psychiatrist his mental institution came from the lazar house, he becomes infuriated" (as cited in Elden, 2023, p. 29).

Foucault argued that the development of modern-day psychiatry and psychology and the emphasis on the classification and diagnosis of mental illnesses was part of an attempt to control the other and force them into a socially acceptable way of life. And did we not accept and succumb to the power of these medical discourses, thus allowing ourselves to be limited by those same discourses? Thus, according to Foucault, what is labeled as "curing" is really a form of domination consequentially from power-knowledge. He questioned our mental health practices, analyzing power in all institutional and structural relations, extending even beyond relationships between people. By exploring the evolution of mental illness and its treatment throughout history, Foucault shed light not only on the history but also on the social and political implications of how we view and treat mental illness today.

Discipline and punish: the birth of the prison (1975)

Discipline and Punish is an exploration of criminality and the history of punishment and discipline in Western societies from the Middle Ages to the modern day. Foucault examined how the methods of punishment have evolved over time, from physical torture and public humiliation to more subtle forms of discipline and control. Before the 18th century, punishments were carried out via ritualistic public executions. The public had its own part to play in the executions, and Foucault described how an audience was necessary for ceremonial punishment. Foucault described, in quite unsettling detail, horrific displays of violence that were a demonstration of the King's power. Over time the people demanded reform. However, lest we jump to thinking we "evolved" or that society "progressed," Foucault believed this call for change derived from outrage over the King's unchecked power more so than from empathy for the tortured criminal.

As public executions became extinct, a new discourse took its place.

> The ideal punishment would be transparent to the crime that it punishes; thus, for him who contemplates it, it will be infallibly the sign of the crime that it punishes; and for him who dreams of the crime, the idea of the offense will be enough to arouse the sign of the punishment.
>
> *(as cited in Foucault, 1995, pp. 104–105)*

Rather than justice being revenge-focused and enacted through torture such as being drawn and quartered, the people in this era proposed that "criminal justice should 'simply punish'" (p. 74). Criminals became symbolic, cautionary tales to deter others from following suit. As a new discourse became dominant, punishments needed to fit the crime, and "Society" no longer wanted to violently punish the body but punish and reform the soul. Although, to my knowledge, this is not mentioned by Foucault, I think of the shaming punishment of Hester Prynne in *The Scarlet Letter*.

Foucault made it clear that just because time progressed, it did not mean *progress*. It did not mean that our methods of punishment progressed; they were just different— actually, in many ways, they had become worse because the methods of punishing were now more subtle. Instead of being put on display for the community, prisoners were kept isolated from society. Prisons had replaced lazar houses. Rather than making the punishment of criminals public, prisons imposed punishment on them within the confines of the prison walls.

Foucault looked at the historical, social, political, and economic knowledge-power dynamics of punishment and how it no longer was short-term and befitting the crime but now a long-term measurement used to maintain social order through means of confinement, which he thought was more about viewing inmates as threatening and quarantining them than it was actually about the crime. Based on his *archaeology*, Foucault argued that punishment served to control behavior rather than reform or rehabilitate offenders. How does solitary confinement, for example, really fit the crime committed? Foucault would argue that it is clearly a form of punishment for lack of conformity to the system in which they are confined.

Prisons put a great emphasis on disciplining individuals: controlling what inmates can eat, when they can exercise, what books they are allowed to read, etc. What was most remarkable to Foucault, however, was how the inmates would take it upon themselves to discipline their own behavior. His inspiration for some of his ideas came from the architecture of Jeremy Bentham's *"Panopticon,"* which was an open prison designed such that inmates could never know whether their guards were watching them, and thus they behaved as though they were always being surveilled. Panopticon comes from the ancient Greek roots PAN (all) + OPTICOS (~to see). For the sake of brevity over a meticulous description of the actual architectural structure, it is designed so guards can always see the prisoners, but prisoners cannot see one another, nor would they know whether the guards were watching them at that moment. In such an environment, the inmates, fearing punishment, would become "docile bodies" who controlled *themselves* out of fear of punishment. Inmates would take it upon themselves to discipline *themselves*: to "stay in their lane," keep their heads down, and not draw attention to themselves.

Foucault fleshed this out further, extending this to all citizens in Western societies. All the masses had become docile bodies who did the work of the government themselves with their constant self-discipline. He saw individuals as being subtly controlled through normalizing practices to prevent being shamed, excluded, isolated, or accused of deviance. It was being subtly taught that nonconformity was something to be feared, not celebrated. To feel ashamed of rather than proud of. Self-regulation or adherence to social standards was the way to avoid this, so *self-discipline* has become rampant even outside of specific institutions.

Illustrating how we have become docile bodies today, speaking largely, we accept that there are cameras surveilling us while we walk down the street, that our internet history is saved, that our phone data is tracked and often sold to third parties, and that applications (i.e., apps) can track our locations. There are now cameras embedded in eyeglasses which are available for purchase by the masses. And we run out to purchase them. We participate in our own oppression. Although, Foucault would have had his problems with the use of the word "oppression," because it conveys a top-down power structure, implying that the institutions oppress the people. However, he wanted to emphasize that it is more of a bottom-up structure, as the people police themselves. For Foucault, the word "oppression" oversimplifies the complex dynamics at work.

Our modern-day society mirrors the Panopticon's molding of docile bodies through self-surveillance, a subtle exercise of power. Again, speaking largely, we are more concerned about buying surveillance devices with good camera quality (i.e., 4K vs. 1080p) than the implications of every eyeglass- and sunglass-wearer documenting our every move. Think about how differently we perform therapy when we are watched or recorded. Even this is a simple example of us policing ourselves to act a certain way to avoid criticism.

At the same time as outlining the history of punishments and how they were carried out, Foucault outlined the history of cultural discourses—understandings of who "deserved" to be punished, disciplined, and controlled. In this book Foucault highlighted the ways we punish and discipline those whom society considers dangerous. The most important questions from his earlier work still resonate: who chooses where the line is between sane and insane, normal and abnormal? We find recurring themes. Discourses are shaped by knowledge-power, and they oppress those who deviate. In the end, it is not just the institutions that oppress us, we also oppress ourselves by policing our own and our neighbors' actions.

DISTILLING FOUCAULT'S CONCEPTS FOR PRACTICAL APPLICATION

In Foucault's *Madness and Civilization*, he discussed *dividing practices* where individuals deemed as a threat to larger society are isolated from the masses in institutions just like lepers were isolated in lazar houses. Due to discourses, individuals are socially "othered" with an ick factor. Further, societal forms of control are justified by reigning discourses. Think, for example, of the discourse of juvenile delinquents needing to be "scared straight" "for their own good." Also, consider the example of setting protective curfews at in-patient facilities for those diagnosed with autism or the more extreme example of locking up labeled schizophrenics or suicidal individuals "to protect them from themselves" and "so they can get better." Like Foucault, my point here is not to argue for or against certain practices, but merely to point out our taken-for-granted knowledges. We are familiar with the phrases "scared straight," "for their own good," etc. because of the place these knowledges have in our Western societal practices. Generally, we assume these actions are right or good, as they are in accordance with dominant discourses. Another example of dividing practices is our treatment of the poor and transient. As someone who has worked therapeutically with this population, I would be remiss to not mention sexual offenders as another example. Most of the sexual offenders I therapeutically worked with were unable to find affordable housing that fit the conditions of not being too close to a school or a park. An unfortunate number of times I have heard people say about sex offenders who are poor and unhoused: "I don't care what happens to them," "they deserve to suffer," or even "they should do us all a favor and die." Again, I use this example not to enter into a debate, but to illustrate how dividing practices of separating out the "icky others" from us are commonplace. Dividing practices are also often tied to and justified by scientific knowledges.

Dividing practices often cross over with another type of objectification based on scientific knowledge (to be read with appropriate skepticism). Here, humans are classified into groups that extract them from individual identities. A person is seen as autistic, schizophrenic, or a sex addict. Since psychiatry became a science, the DSM is widely accepted as scientific fact. These are labels that narrow our view of a person through *totalizing practices* of the *medical gaze*. We can see totalizing practices with sexuality as well. Generally speaking, here in the United States we are taught about sex in schools through sexual education classes. These classes do not focus on pleasure ("Of course not!" you may be thinking—hold on to that thought). Western sex education focuses on a medical explanation of *the body,* not the person, and is usually taught through a heteronormative lens focused on biological reproduction and menstruation. Why do we think this is the correct way? Foucault pointed out Eastern cultures often addressed the pleasure and intimacy of sex, as evinced by the Kama Sutra, which focuses not only on sexual positions but also on desire itself. As Foucault and White would point out, Western reification of science (i.e., Scientification) has eclipsed part of the human experience by viewing the person through a Cartesian dualist's framework where they become a body instead of a human being.

Foucault's concept of *subjectification* emphasizes how power does not have a top-to-bottom construction but rather works from the bottom up: from people's self-monitoring and self-discipline.

> Foucault asserted that "modern power" has become a principal system of social control in contemporary Western culture. This system of social control incites people to enact "normalizing judgment" on themselves and on others in an effort to reproduce specific norms about life and identity. In other words, *people* become accomplices to a system of social control in which they exercise and act upon judgments about life according to established norms about behavior and identity. According to Foucault, these norms have been principally constructed by the professional disciplines (law, medicine, psychology, and so on). This system of social control has significantly displaced a system of social control that subjects people to moral judgment by representatives of state institutions.
>
> *(White, 2007, p. 102)*

When people objectify themselves as subject, an individual takes an active role in their own subjugation, surveilling for normalcy in their ideas, thoughts, and behavior, constantly cross-analyzing the data with societal discourses. Individuals monitor their actions through the *normative gaze* when they ask whether this or that thought or behavior is normal. A client may come in wondering if their attraction to a certain gender or genders is normal. In this case, they are viewing themselves as subject through the normative gaze. Individuals experiencing challenges with eating, typically called eating disorders, objectify and monitor their bodies via the medical gaze while seeing how they measure up against societal standards—the normative gaze. A person diagnosed with anorexia nervosa, more often than not, measures their ideal body shape and weight as is deemed normal or ideal by their cultural standards. Foucault's *Discipline and Punish* challenged our ideas of progress. Yes, corporeal punishment no longer makes up the bulk of our punishment for crimes; however, we end up punishing and disciplining ourselves to fit the mold while "othering" others into places where they are "locked away."

SUMMARY

Michel Foucault was a philosopher with many interests. Foucault was interested in the history of mental illness, the history of medicine, the history of criminality and the penal system, and the history of sexuality. He addressed knowledge-power in Western society. A lover of history, he analyzed different dominant discourses—stories that are so predominant we often mistake them for Truth. His books have us question these discourses and the knowledge(s) we think we know. Readers are enticed to ask themselves, "What is madness?," "What do we as a society do with people who are considered mad?," "What is deviance?," "How do we discipline and punish those who deviate and do not conform?," and "How do we discipline ourselves into becoming docile bodies?" Foucault's ideas are very powerful and resonate across disciplines such as history, education, political science, literature, sociology, psychology, and philosophy. Like many philosophers' works, his books can be difficult to read; however, I encourage you to take your time and read some of Foucault's seminal work (i.e., books and lecture notes) to contemplate what his ideas mean for you as a mental health practitioner.

Foucault was fundamentally against totalizing practices which "thingified" people through political and scientific discourses and turned individuals into piles of organs or even numbers. Dominant discourses reinforce the sovereignty of certain knowledges over others. The discourses and practices delineate what is normal and abnormal.

Madness and Civilization explored the history of mental illness and its treatment. In the early Renaissance, the mad were not separated from the rest of society, nor were they labeled mad in the first place. They were simply fools or people who acted foolishly and accepted, often seen as amusing but not threatening. In the early 1600s, madness could be seen as a part of the human condition. Foucault brought up two literary characters from works written in the early 1600s to illustrate this point: Don Quixote and King Lear. However, by the mid-1600s, madness came to be seen as something to be quarantined and controlled. He reminded readers of the connection here to how society had dealt with lepers. Foucault encouraged his readers to contrast such images of madness as foolishness or part of the human condition to seeing madness as something needing to be confined. Foucault continued his analysis up to the publication of his work in the 1960s, discussing how the modern-day treatment of madness is not "better," nobler, or more evolved. He did not see our treatment of madness as "progress" but as changes through cultural times.

In *Discipline and Punish*, Foucault explained the history of Western society's treatment of those who broke societal rules. He brought readers' awareness to the dominant discourses in a manner that encouraged the readers to question what they knew about truths and knowledge. I do not believe it is unimportant that Foucault opened this book with violence and graphic details about Middle-Age punishments. I see this as an attempt to shock the reader into gratitude that we do not live in such primitive times only to shock them again at the end of his book by implying that our methods of discipline and punishment still exist on that level but are just subtler and less performative. It is not that we have better forms of punishment per se, but it is the case that our punishments are usually not in front of an audience but behind closed doors. Furthermore, self-control out of the ever-present fear that one is being surveilled has become a new way of self-discipline and self-punishment, as the individual now does their own surveilling of themselves in addition to falling under the gaze of larger "Society." I end this paragraph with his famous quote: "Is it surprising that prisons resemble factories, schools, barracks, hospitals, which all resemble prisons?" (1995, p. 228).

Foucault is famously praised as a counter-culture thinker. Foucault's ideas, such as his attention to power-knowledge in institutions and social meaning-making, informed Michael White's culturally aware practice. In the next chapter, I discuss the ways in which Foucault's philosophy applies to the narrative therapy "technique" of externalization.

REFLECTIVE QUESTIONS

1. What is the normative gaze?
2. What is the relationship between power-knowledge, control, "the gaze," and docile bodies?
3. Why does the evolution of punishment in Western societies matter?
4. How might power, knowledge, and discourses affect family therapy clients?
5. What are some consequences of totalizing practices?

Keywords

Power-Knowledge

Discourses

Punishment

Control

Discipline

Normative Gaze

Medical Gaze

Docile Bodies

Panopticon

Dividing Practices

Totalizing Practices

Subjectification

Michel Foucault Post-Test (Inspired by Dr. Perry Zurn in Overthink Podcast, 2022)

1. Has punishment worsened over time?
   a. Punishment has changed over time. Instead of punishment being public, it has moved to being private. Solitary confinement is, essentially, the opposite of the public, dramatic punishments by monarchs Foucault discussed. There are dangers to punishment being "behind the scenes" as well as internalized as something wrong with an individual rather than an individual *did* something.
2. In what ways are we policed in our daily lives?
   a. We are policed constantly. For example, rom traffic cameras, data collector apps, and government or business street cameras.
3. In what ways do we police ourselves and others?
   a. We voluntarily police ourselves, our friends, our acquaintances, and our neighbors through "the gaze." We measure people according to what is "acceptable" and "unacceptable," "normal," and "abnormal," and so on.
4. How do we see dividing practices in our daily lives?
   a. We see examples of dividing practices when we, as a society, "other" unhoused or transient people, queer people, the elderly, people with chronic illness, and so on. There are groups of people who societies inevitably separate as dangerous or "icky." We can counter these dividing practices with curiosity.
5. How can we facilitate curiosity over objectification/thingification?
   a. Part of this process involves recognizing power-knowledge's effects of our subjugation. It necessitates a distance from a modernist view of discourses as Truth. Foucault wants us to be "informed consumers" of our discourses.

MICHEL FOUCAULT: PRIMARY SOURCES

Foucault, M. (1980). 'Body/Power' and 'truth and power.' In C. Gordon (Ed.), *Michel Foucault: Power/Knowledge*. Harvester.

Foucault, M. (1988). *Madness and civilization: A history of insanity in the age of reason* (R. Howard, Trans.). Vintage. (Original work published 1961).

Foucault, M. (1995). *Discipline and punish: The birth of the prison* (A. Sheridan, Trans.). Vintage. (Original work published 1975).

Renowned Sources

Elden, S. (2021). *The early Foucault* (dig. ed.). Polity Press.

Elden, S. (2023). *The archaeology of Foucault* (dig. ed.). Polity Press.

Gutting, G. (2019). *Foucault: A very short introduction* (2nd ed.). Oxford University Press.

Hurley, R. (Ed., Trans). (2020). Introduction. In M. Foucault (Ed.), *The history of sexuality 1: The will to knowledge*. Penguin. (Original work published 1976).

Macey, D. (2019). *The lives of Michel Foucault* (dig. ed.). Verso Books.

Paras, E. (2020). *Foucault 2.0: Beyond power and knowledge*. Other Press, LLC.

Oliver, P. (2010). *Foucault: The key ideas*. McGraw-Hill.

White, M. (2007). *Maps of narrative practice*. W. W. Norton.

White, M. (2012). Scaffolding a therapeutic conversation. In T. Malinen, S. J. Cooper, & F. N. Thomas (Eds.), *Masters of narrative and collaborative therapies: The voices of Andersen, Anderson, and White* (pp. 113–150; dig. ed.). Routledge.

Additional References

Nabulsi, A. (2019). Erotic of the extreme, a philosophical perspective: Foucault's understanding of BDSM. In J. R. Pfeffer (Ed.), Desire, performance, and classification: Critical perspectives on the erotic (pp. 27–35).

Overthink Podcast. (2022, January 18). *Interview with Foucauldians – Dr Perry Zurn* [Video]. YouTube. https://youtu.be/Zw8RjBfdAx8?si=nyY_oYe0GMWUiW4S

Sabot, P. (2023). Michel Foucault in the 1950s: Beyond psychology towards radical ontology. *Theory, Culture, & Society*, 40(1–2), 57–70.

CHAPTER 6

What ideas from Foucault resonated with White?

The path to externalization

....

Remember, as you read through these chapters, you can always return to the Introduction to refresh your memory on the terms you learned such as empiricism, postmodernism, social constructionism, and post-structuralism.

QUESTIONS TO THINK ABOUT

1. What about Foucault's philosophy resonated with Michael White?
2. How are clients affected by power-knowledge?
3. Why is deconstructing social discourses critical to practicing narrative therapy?
4. How do Foucault's ideas connect to White's practice of externalization?

Michael White said that Michel Foucault's ideas were the central influence on the birth and practice of narrative therapy (White, 2012). In a chapter in their seminal work entitled "Story, Knowledge, and Power," White and Epston (1990) discussed Foucault's philosophical contributions in the following sections: "Knowledge and Power as Constitutive" (p. 19), "Power/Knowledge" (p. 21), "Ascending vs. Descending Analysis of Power" (p. 23), "Subjugated Knowledges" (p. 25), and "Alternative Stories and Culturally Available Discourses" (p. 27). Clearly, Foucault's (1975/1995) post-structuralist ideas on power, knowledge, discipline, control, and discourses pervade narrative therapeutic work, making it more politically inclined than the other two post-modern family therapy models in this book.

Allying himself with Foucault, White was interested in effects of power-knowledge, and his therapy model encouraged a focus on institutions' effects on communities, families, and individuals. Inspired by Foucault's interest in "becoming someone else that

DOI: 10.4324/9781003439349-9

you were not in the beginning" (as cited in White, 2011, p. 70), White was interested in cultivating clients' autonomy and creating freedom from limiting discourses (Tilsen, 2021). By paying attention to and building upon clients' subordinated/subjugated discourses (White, 2007), they no longer had to internalize problems as within them.

MICHAEL WHITE'S APPLICATION OF THE FOUCAULDIAN TERM: "THE ARCHAEOLOGY OF KNOWLEDGE"

Foucault's archaeology of knowledge (Foucault, 1973) was a process by which he analyzed antecedent and modern-day, taken-for-granted *knowledges* and revisited words and ideas in their historical context. In alignment with Foucault, White emphasized the process of excavating narratives. He solicited the knowledges that composed clients' stories so he could understand the meaning-making and consequences of the problem.

A social constructionist view, White believed humans do not have direct access to the world. As a Foucauldian, White believed humans act upon knowledge passed down and thrust upon them. As mentioned earlier, the *archaeology of knowledge* is Foucault's term for digging up knowledges of an era, seeing when certain knowledges came into being, and noticing what was taken for granted as Truth. White, solitarily or sometimes with Epston, applied Foucault's archaeological process to a therapeutic context, as illustrated in the following excerpt from a Dulwich Centre video (2018). In this video, Michael White aroused his audience's attention with the archaeology of therapeutic terms.

1. How many of you have *psychological needs*? Can you raise your hand if you have psychological needs? I am not asking you to confess these, okay? But I just would like to know whether you have them or not. I can see many people agreeing. I am not surprised because in Western culture, people have had psychological needs since 1929. Okay? They've been around since 1929, and they're increasingly popular. Today more and more people have psychological needs. (00:10–00:49)
2. How many of you have *relationship dynamics*? Would you raise your hand if you have relationship dynamics? Okay. I'm not surprised at that either because these have been around since the 1960s, or a lot of people have relationship dynamics these days. (1:09–1:26)
3. How many of you have *resources—personal resources*? Okay. These have been around for longer than psychological needs; they've been around for a couple of hundred years or so … (2:06–2:19)

And elsewhere:

4. I know that probably many of you probably have a *human nature*, would you say? Who has a human nature here? Would you raise your hand if you have a human nature? Most of you have a human nature. And more and more people in the world are having a human nature, you know. (Pranas Chile, 2024, 47:09–47:21)

White's humorous tone in these videos belies the seriousness of the topic. White exhumed, perhaps bringing it to people's attention for the first time, examples which demonstrated the construction of knowledge in history. In response to a woman objecting during a conference that she does in fact have psychological needs, White retorted:

But it is also interesting to think about it historically, that if you believe psychological needs do exist, then this becomes a universal understanding that we think is applicable to all people in all cultures, *when it is entirely ethnocentric for you to believe that.*

(Pranas Chile, 51:20–51:32)

White continued,

We do believe we have psychological needs. Now, this understanding shapes our action. It's not neutral in its effects. So the idea that we have psychological needs is cultural and historical, and this idea will shape what we actually do (51:34–51:55) ... I am not trying to suggest the idea of psychological needs is a bad idea, but it is really an *idea.*

(52:40–52:46)

The terms psychological needs, relationship dynamics, and personal resources are "almost never questioned" (Dulwich Centre, 5:15), yet they are socially constructed and, lest we forget, did not always—really ever—*exist.* It can be hard to wrap your head around how something that does not exist has real effects. But these constructions are embedded in culture and the discourses (i.e., narratives) that influence us. As White described during the conference, a lot of the terms we use today started out as metaphors. We reify them over time until they become something we learn to think of as real—"psychological needs" being one clear example.

MICHAEL WHITE'S DESCRIPTION OF "PROBLEM-SATURATED DISCOURSES" IN LANGUAGE

Like Foucault, White recognized the constraining effects societal discourses can have on people's lives. Foucault believed that knowledge was not neutral, a sentiment we see echoed by White in his quote above. If knowledge is not neutral and has real effects, the language in those narratives can alter our lives in tangible ways. Regarding language, we do not simply choose some words over other potentially "equal" descriptions. Therapists need to move beyond seeing language as "just semantics" to properly understand narrative therapy. Informed by Foucault, White believed these societal narratives *shape us* in our practices, our thinking, and thus our constructions of our identities and our possibilities of who we can be.

Language must be viewed from a postmodern, not modern, lens. One must conceptualize language as transformative, not representational. To be "in language" in a narrative therapy session is to participate in an activity of creating discourses (i.e., narratives), challenging discourses (i.e., narratives), and re-authoring discourses (i.e., narratives). Both Foucault and White saw the importance of people being the so-called informed consumers of knowledge/discourse.

Just like Foucault, White impugned unhelpful discourses rather than a person's character, although, to be fair, White incorporated light-hearted humor in contrast to Foucault's often-cited derision. From White's conceptualization, clients come into therapy with a discourse/narrative/story that was termed "problem-saturated" (White

& Epston, p. 4), meaning that moments were strung together across time to create and reinforce problematic myths of an individual's identity. Since problem-saturated stories "allow insufficient space for clients' preferred stories" (p. 14), the problem-saturated discourses are essentially an injunction against a person being free of the problem. A narrative therapy conceptualization, then, is that problem-saturated narratives are the problem, not the person.

As postmodernists often do, White and Epston (1990) debunked objectivity from the start, stressing that there are no facts, only interpretations of what we call "facts." Dominant discourses would always be positioned in a cultural, political context where power was at play. Thus, within this Foucauldian-guided model that highlighted power-knowledge, a therapist could take off their veneer of neutrality and yield their quest for empirical facts. Instead, they could replace this process with conscientious attention to clients' past and present narratives as well as the therapist's role in co-constructing future narratives.

To help my readers understand this on a deeper level, I introduce a popular term in the philosophy of "phenomenology." Phenomenology comes from the ancient Greek roots PHAINOMENON (~something shown) + LOGOS (~to know). Husserl introduced phenomenology as a philosophical study of phenomena in the early 20th century. Qualitative researcher Jonathan Smith introduced a research method called interpretative phenomenological analysis (IPA) over 20 years ago. This qualitative research approach focuses on exploring and interpreting the research participants' "lived experience." The term lived experience refers to a person's experience of their world, rejecting the possibility of an unequivocal, objective understanding of it. To speak of one's lived experience is to speak in a way that treasures their idiosyncratic experiences, history, beliefs, emotions, culture, and context; privileging this over a modernist notion of finding what *really* happened. Narrative therapy's emergence engendered genuine therapeutic interest in people's lived experiences and gave rise to a different way to practice. Narrative therapy is about delving into the client's lived experience and honoring the uniqueness of their experiences and how they choose to tell them.

WHITE'S CONCEPTUALIZATION OF FOUCAULT'S CONCEPT OF "THE OBJECTIFICATION OF INDIVIDUALS"

> Many of the problems that people encounter in life come to represent the "truth" of their identity. For example, in the context of the professional disciplines, it is not uncommon for therapists to refer to a person as "disordered" or "dysfunctional," and in wider culture it is not uncommon for people to consider themselves or others "incompetent" or "inadequate" by nature.
>
> *(White, 2007, pp. 25–26)*

White was certainly deeply affected by Foucault's analysis of the Panopticon described in Chapter 5 (e.g., White, 1991). White noted the danger of the omnipresent normative and medical gazes and the effects on mental health professionals as well as clients. He said, "These knowledges are not about discoveries regarding the 'nature' of persons and of relationship, but are constructed knowledges" (1991, p. 28). We are taught to see problems internalized within individuals. Using Foucauldian terminology, this is an *objectification of individuals* (White, 2007) or, to use White's catchy word for it, a *"thingification"* (White & Epston, 1990) which involves a gaze that ignores individuality and humanity and privileges classification. This process is dehumanizing. "Thingification" is making a person into a thing. The *normative gaze* surveilles individuals to see whether they color inside the lines, so to speak, and it is run by shame and the fear of ostracization. "According to Foucault," White and Epston said, "We live in a society where evaluation or normalizing judgment has replaced the judiciary and torture as a primary mechanism of social control—this is a society of the ever-present 'gaze'" (p. 24).

Foucault's work called attention to the abhorrent ways in which we become objectified or "thingified" in societies. First, we are objectified by the normative gaze by which society determines to what degree certain aspects of our identity and life practices are atypically heinous or accepted as commonplace. Second, we are objectified by the medical gaze by which society objectifies individuals like automatons, seeing people as compilations of brain and bodily functions and dysfunctions. Third and most odious, we objectify ourselves as *docile bodies*, becoming both the prisoner and warden as we monitor our every move.

In a therapeutic context, we might see evidence of clients being affected by the normative gaze when they ask whether their sexual inclinations are normal. We can observe effects of the medical gaze if a client says they are unable to have a relationship because they "are Borderline"—referring to borderline personality disorder (BPD). We can notice a client's Panopticon-like surveillance with clients who avoid eating to look slimmer (White, 1991).

The medical gaze

The *medical gaze* regards individuals not as distinct persons but rather as an assembly of bodily tissues, organs, cells, and molecules. White knew the medical gaze, "which totalizes the person's experience" (Fernandez et al., 2023, p. 273), leads to discrimination, marginalization, and oppression (White, 2007) in the name of science. Further, White took a non-expert, non-pathologizing stance to avoid perpetuating oppression through the medical gaze. He was openly critical of psychotherapeutic work which encouraged the objectification of individuals, examples of which may include narratives such as, "Jordan has self-esteem problems" or "Jamie is depressed" (Robertson et al., 2023). And he reminded us, from a Foucauldian standpoint, "A domain of knowledge is a domain of power" (White, 1991, p. 27). Although a marked improvement, White would also not likely have said, "Jordan is *experiencing* self-esteem problems" or "Jamie is *experiencing* depression," since both of those conceptualizations assume the existence of "Self-Esteem Problems" or "Depression" which still reinforces the medical gaze.

As well-known narrative therapists Jill Freedman and Gene Combs described a therapist's predicament:

> Health insurers require a DSM diagnosis, and all the major, "legitimate" DSM diagnoses are individually based. Even in a small private therapy practice, to

be paid for our work we must conceptualize people's problems as disorders in individual bodies. We must measure the families we see according to individualistic, biologically based norms. We are pushed to diagnose people as though the labels derived from such norms define their identities, and to file pathology-based reports to justify each hour or portion thereof we spend in following ever-more-rigidly defined practices.

(Combs & Freedman, 2016, p. 212)

Identities being central to narrative therapy, recall White emphasizing there is no such thing as "psychological needs," etc. Psychological needs do not exist other than as a construction in language. What he would have said would likely be a question instead of a statement. What I believe he might have asked is, "Jordan, what do you think the problem is?" He might secondarily have asked, "What effects has this problem had on your life?"

The first step in practicing narrative therapy is to have awareness that labels like "psychological needs," "self-esteem problems," and "depression" are socially constructed. The second step is to challenge those social constructs. This inherently involves separating the person from the problem, because you sincerely do not believe the person is or has a problem. They are simply experiencing life. Some clients find relief in that idea alone.

The third is to continue to be conscientious of the language used, acknowledging that the language the therapist uses creates a reality for both client and therapist. A narrative therapist aims not to perpetuate limiting discourses or narratives.

Often, new therapists think about the language coming from the client. Here, in narrative therapy, there is responsibility on the therapist to be cautious about their own language. As a narrative therapist, you are helping the client shape their reality differently. That takes a lot of commitment to the idea that language is constructive. White believed none of these labels are "real" on their own, but language makes them real. Thus, in a way, nothing is real until language makes it real.

Personal agency

Rather than reifying expert knowledge, White approached narrative therapy with an "irreverent, maverick spirit" (Epston et al., 2019, p. 7) that aimed to cultivate *personal agency*: "that sense of being able to regulate one's own life; to intervene in one's life to affect its course according to one's intentions, and to do this in ways that are shaped by one's knowledges of life" (White & Morgan, 2006, p. 40). To achieve this outcome, White more or less performed surgical operations on internalized narratives and brought them outward for analysis. He called this *"deconstruction,"* carefully noting that his use of the word did not fully align with that of its philosophical originator and Foucault's contemporary, Jacques Derrida (White, 1991).

"Foucault argued for the 'insurrection' of the subjugated knowledges against the 'institutions and against the effects of the knowledge and power that invent scientific discourse'" (White & Epston, p. 27). Thus, to preserve clients' agency, White argued therapists need to increase their own attention to their therapeutic position of power and their part within each institutionalized power-knowledge system. Therefore, it would be antithetical to say something like, "If the client doesn't change, they are not ready to do the work." This conceptualization takes away from the responsibility the therapist has in the therapeutic relationship. White was very conscientious of his being in a position of power in relation to the client. He did not want to perpetuate the hierarchy by lording over his expert power-knowledge as one who *fixes* people. In White's model, people are not broken. The view of people as broken would refer back to the medical gaze which sees people through a dehumanized lens of a bunch of organs and brain waves not functioning correctly rather than as complex, diverse, and unique individuals.

Knowledge-power

Allying with Foucault, Michael White believed power plays a fundamental role in shaping and influencing clients' lives and that individuals become active participants in a system of societal regulation (White, 2007). White and Epston recapitulated:

> Rather than proposing that this form of power represses, Foucault argued that it subjugates. It forges persons as "docile bodies" and conscripts them into activities that support the proliferation of "global" and "unitary" knowledges [and the] "objective reality" knowledges of the modern scientific disciplines (p. 20).

Quoting and elaborating upon Foucault, White and Epston addressed how individuals are subjugated by knowledge-power and its claims on truth. As the founders explained, we are ensnared in a complex network:

> Foucault thus dissuades us from a concern with an "internal point of view" for the explanation of the operation of power, challenging any preoccupations we might have with who intends its effects and what decisions are made about its exercise. Since we are all caught up in a net or web of power/knowledge, it is not possible to act apart from this domain, and we are simultaneously undergoing the effects of power and exercising this power in relation to others. However, this does not, by any means, suggest that all persons are equal in the exercise of power, nor that some do not suffer its subjugating effects very much more than others.
>
> *(White & Epston, p. 22)*

There are many discourses we can point to, some more helpful than others. In White's practice, he encouraged the development of the *subordinated (or subjugated) discourses*—discourses that haven't had the space to grow because dominant discourses have taken over. For example, a client of mine said, "How do I know if I am being a good partner if my partner and I do not get married?" This client has been affected by the discourse that marriage is a necessary step in solidifying a committed relationship. Additionally, the dominant discourse has made her believe that marriage is an objective measure of how "well" she is doing in her relationship. You can also see she has been affected by discourses that define what a good partner is.

The *subjugated discourse* is a narrative that does not follow the mainstream, dominant discourse. Subjugated discourses are stories that have been overlooked by the client. While the client was consumed with thinking about how to be a good partner, marriage as an objective measure, and of marriage being a necessary step in a committed relationship; she was depriving herself of possibilities to create new identities for herself. The exact subjugated discourse (or narrative) does not matter as much as it is *a* subjugated discourse (or narrative) brought to light.

The client had inadvertently limited her identity of who she is, what her role is, how she should live, and so on. By exploring subjugated discourses, the narrative therapist helps the client "connect the dots" of their experience in different ways (i.e., *re-authoring*). After deconstructing the dominant discourse and re-authoring, the client can build upon their unique story of strengths and alternative identities.

Re-authoring is different than reframing. In reframing, you present a new way to look at a person, problem, or situation. In re-authoring, you are asking questions such that the individual on their own comes to see a person, problem, situation, or opportunities differently. Re-authoring is co-writing a new story, building upon the subjugated narratives. Reframing is re-presenting based on exceptions, not necessarily collaboratively creating and exploring something new.

To apply these concepts of dominant narratives, subjugated narratives, reframing, and re-authoring, let us look at another example. Marielle is a White American client who identifies as non-binary and uses they/them pronouns; however, Marielle is subjected to the dominant discourse and normative gaze that view gender as a binary. The dominant narrative is that people are either male or female. Marielle's non-binary identity can be considered a subjugated narrative, as it goes against the dominant discourse. Whereas a solution focused brief therapist might say, "Marielle, how have you been able to have the tenacity to keep going through all these obstacles?"; a narrative therapist might say, "It seems society is telling you who you are and who you can be. 'Where do you stand on this'?" (White, 2005, p. 5). The first gives Marielle a label of a tenacious person and invites Marielle to build upon it with times they have demonstrated tenacity. The second refuses the temptation to label, even positively, and co-authors with Marielle to see how Marielle wants to describe their identity.

Docile bodies

Recall Foucault's belief that society forges docile bodies. To Foucault, we have all become docile bodies who police ourselves to see whether we fall within the parameters of "normal" and work to correct the ways in which we might stray. White was clearly affected by Foucault's description of the Panopticon and the effects of surveillance (e.g., 1991), where individuals play "an active role in their own subjugation" (White & Epston, p. 24). For example, White (1991) detailed the case of "Amy." Amy was a 23-year-old woman whose presenting problem was anorexia nervosa. Pay close attention to how White described her case of self-surveillance and listen for similarities with the Panopticon:

> I first reviewed the effects anorexia nervosa was having in the various domains of her life—including the social, the emotional, the intellectual, and, of course,

the physical. I wasn't surprised to learn that it had her constantly comparing herself to others, and that it had instilled in her a sense that she was being perpetually evaluated by others. Apart from this, it was enforcing a shroud of secrecy around her life and isolating her from others. Predictably, it was requiring her to watch over herself, to police herself. It had her engaging in operations on her own body, attempting to forge it into a shape that might be considered acceptable—a "docile body." And it had her punishing her own body for its transgressions. I then engaged Amy in an investigation of how she had been recruited into these various practices, procedures and attitudes; these "disciplines of the self" according to gendered specifications for personhood; this hierarchical and disciplinary attitude and relationship to her own body.

(White, 1991, p. 23)

Amy's situation connects back to Foucauldian concepts of the medical gaze, the normative gaze, and docile bodies. She dealt with many doctors as a patient diagnosed with anorexia, and each treated her in accordance with what the medical textbooks would say according to her Body Mass Index (BMI) and so on. She also was clearly affected by the normative gaze, where society's expectations of a woman to look a certain way changed her relationship to herself and her own body. Finally, she monitored her body and what she ate as a form of "discipline" and "control." By trying to conform to certain standards, she was essentially working against herself.

Notice how rather than label Amy an anorexic, White used the language: "I first reviewed *the effects anorexia nervosa was having* in the various domains of her life." This again demonstrates his belief that the problem is the problem; the person is not the problem. This is a clear example of externalization—un-"thingifying" Amy.

Externalization

Externalization is a process of moving from objectification of people to an objectification of the problem. In their book *Narrative Means to Therapeutic Ends,* White and Epston (1990) explained: "Externalizing is an approach to therapy that encourages persons to objectify and, at times, to personify the problems that they experience as oppressive" (p. 38). In other words, the problem is objectified, not the person; therefore, the therapist and the client are in collaboration, processing the problem. We must remind ourselves that people are not inherently problematic, and no label can actually describe a whole person. When we concretize a person as "x," we often limit who they can become. Again, White objectified the problem of anorexia, not the person of Amy as "an anorexic."

As White and Epston said,

Externalization is helpful in the interruption of the habitual reading and performance of unhelpful stories. As persons become separated from their stories, they are able to experience a sense of personal agency; as they break from their performance of their stories, they experience a capacity to intervene in their own lives and relationships (p. 16).

Externalization leads to personal agency and empowerment on the part of the client. And it requires culpability, accountability, and responsibility on the part of the therapist.

The main point of this chapter is that externalization is more than a technique. *Externalizing conversations* are just that—conversations. It is not a "technique" that one applies simply by using a metaphor (White, 2007). The metaphor is picked with foresight, introduced with purpose, and is used throughout the therapeutic session or sessions. Although there are different things one can choose to externalize, typically, a practitioner will stick with one main one, making sure it separates the person from the problem. The thing externalized should fit with both the therapist and client and go against the objectification of the client, bringing Foucault's ideas of combatting oppression to the forefront.

Foucault's philosophy is central to picking what to externalize and how. A narrative therapist should recall Foucault's cautions of viewing people through society's normative gaze, through science's medical gaze, or encouraging an individual's self-surveillance and cultivation of "docile bodies." To conceptualize externalization as an isolated family therapy technique misses the mark by extracting it from its context—what White did AND why he did it. In other words, not just any old metaphor will do. And you need to know where you are going when you introduce the metaphor.

Externalizing internalized discourses

Externalization is used to undo the "thingification" of people instilled by those pesky dominant discourses and can be used in any situation since all therapeutic conversations are situated in language and in culture. Because the problem is located outside of the person,

> Externalizing conversations can provide an antidote to these understandings by objectifying the problem. They employ practices of objectification of the problem against cultural practices of objectification of people. This makes it possible for people to experience an identity that is separate from the problem; the problem becomes the problem, not the person.
>
> *(2007, p. 9)*

Some famous examples of White's externalization work with children are "sneaky poo" for encopresis (White & Epston), "special friend" for ADHD (White, 1991), and "the naughty little phobia" for a gastro/intestinal food phobia (White & Morgan).

Examples of externalization

Let's look at one of White's most famous cases:

Andrew: Okay. As I'm sure you've guessed, we've been having a really hard time with Jeffrey. He's got ADHD. This has now been confirmed by two pediatricians and an educational psychologist.

Beth: We're only just learning about ADHD.

M: So the diagnosis is pretty recent?

Beth: We've known for sure since the start of this year—that's about 8 or 9 months.

M: What's it been like to have this diagnosis?

Beth: It's been quite a relief, hasn't it Andrew?

Andrew: Yeah, we are both relieved to at least have a name for it.

M: Making diagnoses is not my specialty.

Andrew: But surely you have seen a lot of this, and you'd be able to …

M: Yes, I have seen a lot of children who have been diagnosed with ADHD. But my work with them has not involved me making this diagnosis.

Andrew: Are you serious? Are you really serious? *(turning to Beth)* So just what are we going to do next?

M: I do have an idea about how we might find out what sort of ADHD is giving you all such a difficult time.

Beth: *(with a "this looks promising" expression on her face)* Okay, let's hear it.

M: All right then Jeffrey, tell me this. Just tell me this one thing. What color is your ADHD?

Jeffrey: *(momentarily bewildered and turning to his parents, who both shrug; then turning back to me)* Dunno.

M: Ah-hah! I knew it! Now I know why Jeffrey's ADHD is just free to run around upsetting everything. How could Jeffrey do anything to stop this if he doesn't even know what his ADHD looks like? Jeffrey, how could you do anything about what your ADHD is up to? (White, 2007, pp. 11–14)

Right away, White jumped into separating ADHD from the identified patient/client, Jeffrey. Instead of objectifying Jeffrey, White "thingified" the ADHD. Rather than assume an expert stance of knowing about ADHD, White adopted a non-expert, stance, talking about his experience with children who had already been diagnosed. By doing so, he separated himself from the medical gaze and embodied a non-pathologizing stance. Notice how White used the language of *diagnosis* rather than say something like, "What has it been like to finally figure out what's *wrong* with Jeffrey?" Pay attention to how White has already externalized so close to the start of the session, using the phrase "ADHD is giving you all such a difficult time." By saying "you all," he is also avoiding singling out Jeffrey as the problem, and he is moving to a relational conceptualization where the family can come together to support each other when ADHD "plays tricks" on their lives (p. 20).

The next example is from White and Morgan (2006). Here White is working with a different child, combining art therapy with narrative therapy.

I fetched some art materials, and Richard went to work. I peered over his shoulder as he did so, and as these fears began to take shape it took my breath away to see what Richard had been struggling with. These were indeed very scary fears, and I observed:

M: No-one who had fears like this running around in their lives would be able to get any sleep at all!

Richard: Well, I hardly get any sleep myself!

M: Well, is that fair?

Richard: What?

M: Do you think it is fair that these fears take away your sleep?

Richard: No, it's not fair. It's really not fair....

Richard: Something just has to be done about this. These fears need a good education.

M: Oh, so a good education would...

Richard: Fix things, yeah ...

M: Okay. Great! ...

Richard: They shouldn't be allowed just to run around all over the place at night.

M: I reckon you could be right about that (pp. 3–5)

By starting the therapeutic conversation this way, White immediately set to work on externalization, separating the person from the problem: separating Richard from his fears. Instead of characterizing Richard as a fearful boy, White externalized the fears and validated their scariness. Asking whether it is "fair" aligns with Foucault's emphasis on discourses as subjugating, and we see White encouraging Richard to cultivate his own voice. As the conversation progressed naturally, it was Richard, not even White, who made the suggestion to do something to the problem: "to reeducate" the problem. The problem-saturated story was reworked such that Richard had a relationship to the problem as though it were outside of him. This is the process of externalizing internalized discourses.

Keep in mind, you do not have to come up with the most brilliant, perfect metaphor. With externalization, try not to get caught up in the idea that you need to externalize depression as a blue monster or rainy cloud. Narrative therapist Alice Morgan (2002) externalized simply by adding "the" before the presenting problem. For example, "The Depression" or "The Anxiety." This allows the client to see themselves having a relationship to the problem without the problem being a part of them or defining who they are. If you adopt a Foucauldian lens and view someone as a human who is being negatively affected by certain social discourses which trick them into thinking something is wrong with them, you can subtly use language such that externalizing conversations happen naturally.

Deconstruction is the process of breaking down discourses, and this process is tied to externalization.

It is quite common for this unraveling process to reveal the history of the "politics" of the problems that bring people to therapy. This is a history of the power relations that people have been subject to and that have shaped their negative conclusions about their life and their identity. This unraveling (i.e., deconstruction) deprives these conclusions of a "truth" status and calls them into question. As an outcome, people find that their lives are no longer tied to these negative conclusions, and this puts them in a position to explore other territories of their lives. In these explorations, they invariably arrive at more positive conclusions about their identity. I have found this sort of unraveling or deconstruction of people's negative conclusions about life to be a very helpful aspect of externalizing conversations.

(White, 2007, p. 27)

This can look like asking questions about the client's values and where they came from such as, "What is a good mother?" and "Where did you learn that idea from?" As Morgan said, "These conversations examine some of the 'taken for granted' ideas that influence people's views" (2002, p. 88).

To "properly" "do" externalization, first consider deconstruction. Think about Society and the systems and institutions that perpetuate the dominant societal discourses. Consider how these discourses subjugate our personal narratives. Think about deconstructing as unpacking discourses so as to be "informed consumers" of these narratives we are buying into. Practitioners can tap into a post-structuralist rebellious position, poking at discourses and asking questions about societal values and ideas, perpetuated by institutions that may be harming clients. The emphasis for the narrative therapist *"should"* be to use language wisely to (1) separate the client from the problem and (2) unpack the discourse to see if it is one the client truly agrees with. This deconstruction-externalization is the Foucauldian heart of narrative therapy. White and Epston believed these externalizing conversations allowed for other opportunities for a new story. As the narrative therapist continues their externalizing conversations, they are re-authoring with the client. The cultivation of the individual's identity comes naturally as clients get more of a say in their own life and what they want and do not want.

SUMMARY

White and Epston's narrative therapy model relies on Foucault's post-structuralist ideas such as knowledge-power and its effects on our social discourses. Certain practices of power are favored, while the others are set aside. Thus some knowledges earn the societal ribbon of "fact" while other knowledges are marginalized. Recall White's focus on ethnocentrism in his response to the conference attendee. There is no denying a political, cultural, and history epicenter in narrative therapy.

Narrative therapists focus on deconstruction, the unraveling of discourses, and externalization, the separation of the person from the problem. Like the miracle question in solution focused brief therapy (SFBT), externalization is the buzzword that many therapists take away from the model without understanding fully *what it is* and *why it is used*. Do not fall into the trap of thinking that externalization is just a metaphor; it must be applied in a particular way in order to "un-thingify" the person. The metaphor is carefully chosen as an option to rid the person of "oppressive*" discourse (see Chapter 5). White and Epston's work focused on freeing clients for more possibilities through externalizing *conversations*, so externalization is not a technique you apply once and stop. If you believe these Foucauldian ideas about power-knowledge and its effects on communities and individuals, you will be inclined to provide alternative discourses for clients to liberate them from the problem—not necessarily "solve" the problem. Consider that perhaps there is no problem to be solved, and the problem is merely that the person believes they (or others) are the problem. Alternatively, consider a problem like Jeffrey's ADHD, where a problem has a relationship to a person but *is not* the person. These beliefs compose externalizing conversations. If you wish to work on externalization, work to understand Foucault's ideas about docile bodies and how we might undo deleterious effects to the best of our ability.

REFLECTIVE QUESTIONS

1. How do you see Michael White's narrative therapy approach as different from diagnostic approaches?
2. In the example, how might Richard be empowered through narrative therapy?
3. How do Michel Foucault's ideas on power, knowledge, and discourses inform White's practice of externalization?
4. Reflect on White's practice of separating the person from the problem. How might this be applied in non-therapeutic contexts as well?

Keywords

Dominant Narrative/Dominant Story
Subjugated Narrative/Subjugated Story
Externalization
Deconstruction
Re-Authoring/Re-Storying

Externalization Post-Test (Inspired by White, 2007)

1. How important is "Society" in shaping our beliefs about our identity?
   a. Both Foucault and Michael White emphasize the significant role Society plays in shaping our identities. Power-knowledge related to institutions, discourses, and social norms (re) shape our identities and behaviors. Similarly, White thought social discourses and narratives impacted "negative identity conclusions" (p. 26).
2. Briefly, what do externalizing conversations do?
   a. White said that externalizing conversations "facilitate the unraveling of negative identity conclusions, which deprives these conclusions of a 'truth' status and calls them into question" (p. 27). By engaging in externalizing conversations, you are separating the person from the problem, making room for preferred narratives and positive identity conclusions.
3. When I engage in a deconstructing/externalizing conversation, how do I avoid imposing my own power-knowledge/discourses/narratives on the client?
   a. "Stay in your lane," so to speak, and remember your role as a narrative therapist is like an "*investigative reporter*" in that you do not problem-solve and do not encourage clients to problem-solve (pp. 27–28). In narrative therapy, like in SFBT, you do not problem-solve; however, in narrative therapy, unlike in SFBT, you gather as much detail as you can about the problem and the discourses surrounding it. You can jointly call things into question, but avoid offering your new "truth" to replace theirs. This latter aspect certainly differs from SFBT where you may offer a reframe to do exactly that. I believe narrative therapy is more similar to collaborative-dialogic practice (C-DP) in that you are hesitant to highlight anything as true, right, or real, believing instead that asking questions can be more beneficial than providing answers.

4. How will I know what metaphor to use?

    a. Quickly identifying a useful metaphor will become easier with practice. When you listen to a client, you are listening for the discourses that are affecting their life as well as unique outcomes that can lead you to preferred narratives. Remain aware of how your client describes their problem and recall Foucault's ideas about subjugation. For new learners, it is often helpful to attune to what metaphors *not* to use. White said, "I do not introduce battle metaphors and do not initiate a totalizing of the problem. When people embrace a singular fight metaphor, I remain alert to other metaphors that might be employed in describing action or proposals for action in the revision of the person's relationship to the problem. Remaining alert to the emergence of other metaphors allows for the possibility of gradually focusing on something other than 'the fight' (p. 37)." If you are looking for the basics, you may consider using Alice Morgan as a resource, whose works can be found in the references at the end of this chapter. Watching Michael White's conferences on YouTube (or another platform) has been immensely helpful for me to see how Foucault ties directly into externalization, making it easier for me to determine which metaphors would be most and least useful. The more you can hear White talk about totalizing practices, dividing practices, the Panopticon, docile bodies, and "the gaze," the easier it will be for you to make these connections in practice.

5. What if I have a client who already has a severe mental health diagnosis such as schizophrenia? What does externalization look like then?

    a. White (2007) encouraged what he called a "cool engagement" over a "hot engagement" and provided an example of his interaction with a schizophrenic client: "I met with Harold, who expressed a primary concern about the harassment that the hostile voices were subjecting him to. The externalizing conversation that developed in relationship to this did not encourage a hot engagement with these voices. It did not encourage Harold to confront the voices, discipline them, or wrestle with them in any way. Rather, Harold was encouraged to characterize these voices by typifying the way that they spoke, by describing the tactics of power they used to establish dominance, by identifying the strategies that they employed to establish themselves as an authority on the motives of others, and by determining the agendas and the purposes that were expressed in all of this" (p. 28). White continued to describe how the metaphors the therapist chooses will be based on the descriptions of the problem. "For example, if people characterize the influence of the problem as oppressive, the second-phrase postures will be oppositional, and people will take action to 'liberate' their lives from the problem. If people characterize this influence as unjust, the posture assumed will be a moral one. If people characterize this influence to be uninformed, a teaching posture will be assumed, and action will be taken to educate the problem about what is in the best interest of people's lives" (p. 30).

MICHEL FOUCAULT AND MICHAEL WHITE: PRIMARY SOURCES

White, M. (1991). Deconstruction and therapy. *Dulwich Centre Newsletter, 3,* 21–40.
White, M. (2005). *Workshop notes.* www.dulwichcentre.com.au
White, M. (2007). *Maps of narrative practice.* W. W. Norton.

White, M. (2011). *Narrative practice: Continuing conversations*. W. W. Norton.

White, M. (2012). Scaffolding a therapeutic conversation. In T. Malinen, S. J. Cooper, & F. N. Thomas (Eds.), *Masters of narrative and collaborative therapies: The voices of Andersen, Anderson, and White* (pp. 113–150, dig. ed.). Routledge.

White, M., & Epston, D. (1990). *Narrative means to therapeutic ends*. W. W. Norton.

White, M., & Morgan, A. (2006). *Narrative therapy with children and their families*. Dulwich Centre Publications.

Renowned Sources

Combs, G., & Freedman, J. (2016). Narrative therapy's relational understanding of identity. *Family Process, 55,* 211–224.

Dulwich Centre Foundation: Narrative Therapy. (2018, April 4). *Michael White, narrative therapist: Funny moments* [Video]. YouTube. https://youtu.be/TT73fQVvya8?si=M1VYXcaPpmX4DNle

Epston, D., Carlson, T. S., & polanco, m. (2019). Re-imagining narrative therapy: An ecology of magic and mystery for the maverick. *Journal of Narrative Family Therapy, 3,* 1–18.

Foucault, M. (1973). *The order of things: An archaeology of the human sciences*. Vintage Books.

Foucault, M. (1995). *Discipline and punish: The birth of the prison* (A. Sheridan, Trans.). Vintage. (Original work published 1975).

Morgan, A. (2002). Beginning to use a narrative approach in therapy. *International Journal of Narrative Therapy and Community Work, 1,* 85–90.

Pranas Chile. (2024). Prácticas Narrativas para el Trabajo con las Consecuencias del Trauma [Narrative Practices for Working with the Consequences of Trauma]. https://pranaschile.org/videos

Additional References

Fernandez, K. T. G., Martin, A. T. M. B., & Ledesma, D. A. S. (2023). The use of narrative therapy on paranoid schizophrenia. *Psychological Studies, 68,* 273–280.

Robertson, C., Clegg, G., & Huntley, J. (2023). *Storytelling in medicine: How narrative can improve practice* (2nd ed.). CRC Press.

Tilsen, J. (2021). *Queering your therapy practice: Queer theory, narrative therapy, and imagining new identities*. Routledge.

PART IV

Solution Focused Brief Therapy

CHAPTER 7

An introduction to solution focused brief therapy

....

Remember, as you read through these chapters, you can always return to the Introduction to refresh your memory on the terms you learned such as empiricism, modernism, social constructionism, post-structuralism, and epistemology.

QUESTIONS TO THINK ABOUT

1. Why might sessions be called "interviews" and therapists be called "coaches" in SFBT?
2. In what ways does an SFBT practitioner use the client's expertise?
3. What information is the most important to SFBT practitioners?
4. In what ways does an SFBT therapist use language that may seem unusual?

Insoo Kim Berg, a Korean-born Wisconsinite and social worker, married fellow Milwaukeean Steve de Shazer, a professional saxophonist and social worker (Durrant, 2007; Pichot, 2014). Berg and de Shazer met while studying brief, strategic practices at the Mental Research Institute (MRI) in Palo Alto, where their mentor, John Weakland, introduced them in 1977 (De Jong, 2019; Visser, 2013). There they were influenced by Bateson, Erickson, Jackson, Weakland, and Haley (De Jong; de Shazer, 1982; Reiter, 2017) who focused on cybernetics, communication, and identifying failed solution attempts (Berg & Szabó, 2005). Together, this dynamic couple founded solution focused brief therapy (SFBT) in the 1980s (Macdonald, 2011).

Berg and de Shazer left California and created the Milwaukee Brief Family Therapy Center (BFTC) in 1978 (Berquez & Jeffery, 2024; Macdonald, 2016). Their original team at the BFTC included Yvonne Dolan, Eve Lipchik, Gale Miller, and Elam Nunally (Dolan, 2024, p. x), and they often saw working class clients struggling with substance

DOI: 10.4324/9781003439349-11

use and transience (Dolan). Berg and de Shazer reoriented their work from simply *brief* to *solution-focused* in 1982 (Lee, 2011). Given their history at MRI where it was encouraged not to surpass 10 sessions (Kim, 2013), it is unsurprising that Berg and de Shazer co-developed a brief model. Given their population's needs, it is unsurprising that they created a solution-oriented model. What *is* surprising, however, is SFBT's intense future-focus.

SFBT is not just about solutions; it is about replacing the past with the future as the locus of therapy. Although entirely distinct from narrative therapy, SFBT does borrow a story metaphor "since [stories] shape people's goals and expectations [for the future]" (Miller et al., 1991, p. 315). SFBT recalibrates to how to create the better future a client describes—*not the future a therapist has in mind for the client* (Froerer et al., 2018). SFBT is a brief, solution-oriented, and future-focused postmodern family therapy model.

AN INDUCTIVE, EMPIRICAL APPROACH

SFBT practice alleges it was formed based on research about what worked therapeutically, prior to adherence to a theory, so it is described as being created *inductively* as opposed to deductively (de Shazer et al., 2021). However, one might argue that the BFTC therapists were already influenced by systems theory and cybernetics from their MRI training, which percolated into their SFBT work; therefore, it may be more fair to say SFBT evolved inductively *and* deductively. After all, even if their theory evolved, this does not mean that no theory ever existed *a priori* (Latin: "from what is before").

It is the norm to highlight SFBT as an inductive model, but I do not want my readers to fall into the assumption that "inductive" is synonymous with "pragmatic." Neither should "inductive" be thought of as more research-based. Inductive and deductive are simply two different ways to reason to a conclusion.

> In philosophy, deductive arguments are sometimes illustrated by providing an example in which an argument's premises logically entail its conclusion. For example: Socrates is a man. All men are mortal. Therefore, Socrates is mortal. By contrast, inductive arguments are said to be those that make their conclusions merely probable. They might be illustrated by an example like the following: Most Greeks eat olives. Socrates is a Greek. Therefore, Socrates eats olives. Assuming the truth of those premises, it is likely that Socrates eats olives, but that is not guaranteed. According to this view, this latter argument is inductive.
> *(Internet Encyclopedia of Philosophy, 2024, para. 3–8)*

"In research, inductive approaches move from specific to general while deduction begins with the general and ends with the specific" (Soiferman, 2010, p. 3). With SFBT, inductive is the widely accepted descriptor since their new approach in the 1980s was grounded in empiricism. As you will recall from the Introduction, empirical research is a form of modernist research based upon observation. Sessions at the BFTC were witnessed live behind a one-way mirror and the therapist would consult the team behind the mirror[1] (Kim); meanwhile, detailed notes were kept on "therapists' questions, statements, or behaviors that led to clients reporting positive outcomes" (Dolan, p. 3). That SFBT was founded upon empirical (i.e., modernist) research is a pretty unusual start for a *post*modern model. This goes back to SFBT being a bridge model, as explained in the Introduction.

EVIDENCE-BASE

SFBT prides itself on being an evidence-based model (Kim et al., 2019). Peter De Jong and Berg's later research (2002) reported "an improvement rate of 74% versus the average of 66%" (as cited in Anderson, 2015, p. 198). The practitioner-researchers also concluded that therapy was helpful even in a short number of sessions based on client self-report (De Jong): "Data indicated 80 to 90 percent of therapy was less than 20 sessions; yet most clients said that therapy was useful" (p. 3). Kim (2013, p. 3) reported that clients stayed "an average of 6–10 sessions regardless of the therapist's modality." These research conclusions reinforce the assumption that brief therapy is helpful and that SFBT is a model that can generate positive therapeutic outcomes.

BECOMING KNOWN AS A POSTMODERN, SOCIAL CONSTRUCTIONIST MODEL

As Berg and de Shazer continued their work, they became additionally influenced by postmodern ideas. de Shazer was particularly influenced by the philosophical ideas of Ludwig Wittgenstein (Dolan; Visser), who was not technically postmodern, social constructionist, nor even fully constructivist, although he more closely aligned with linguistic constructivism (see de Shazer, 1991). Regardless, Wittgenstein is a renowned influence on the postmodern, constructivist, and social constructionist philosophical movements (Chenail et al., 2020). Wittgenstein will be discussed in depth in the next chapter.

Wittgenstein's ideas took hold of de Shazer. As de Shazer discovered and became engrossed in Wittgensteinian philosophy, he shared the ideas with Berg and seemingly anyone who would listen (de Shazer et al.). Over time, de Shazer became increasingly influenced by the language-oriented philosopher, and SFBT became increasingly influenced by Wittgenstein's emphasis on language as an *activity* that people do together (de Shazer & Berg, 1992). de Shazer resonated with the later-Wittgensteinian idea that language is not representational of our world and instead is creative. This is certainly a social constructionist aspect: viewing language as constructive of our world rather than representational of it.

As Kim (2013) described, "SFBT *currently* aligns itself more under the metatheory of social constructionism, which asserts that individual constructs are shaped through conversations with others" (p. 6). As a social constructionist model (Bannink), SFBT therapist pays meticulous attention to language (de Shazer & Berg). The postmodern crux of SFBT is using language to empower clients in cooperative conversations (Berg, 1994). I want you, dear reader, to see that SFBT does not have to be as structured as you might find on a website's overview. But there are some necessary language tweaks.

Interestingly, at the beginning of therapy, a solution focused therapist will find it useful to try to help the client shift from using the verb "to be" to the verb "to feel" when talking about the problem while at the end of therapy, when talking about solutions, the therapist will find it useful to help the client make the reverse shift in the verb used to describe the situation.

(de Shazer, 1997, p. 141)

Instead of "I am" it becomes "I feel" and at the end, you switch back from "I feel" to "I am." For example, "I am irresponsible" becomes "I feel irresponsible," and by the end of therapy "I feel responsible" becomes "I am responsible." I endearingly refer to de Shazer's process as *trapping your clients into positives* because you are structuring the language such that it does not give clients a chance to be negative about themselves— linguistically speaking. Language is everything in this model, as will become clearer in the next two chapters. One word can change an entire meaning, as illustrated by de Shazer's move from the word "disease" to "dis-ease" (1991, p. 6).

THE PRACTICE OF SFBT

According to Trepper and colleagues (2013), some "ingredients" for SFBT practice are: (1) putting the locus of a conversation on the client's concerns and preferred future, (2) reframing and cooperatively changing meaning(s), and (3) "inviting clients to co-construct a vision of a preferred future and draw on their past successes, strengths, and resources to make that vision a reality" (p. 16). SFBT practice encourages a good rapport and purposeful solution-focus (Lipchik & de Shazer, 2017). SFBT also borrows from collaborative-dialogic practice (C-DP) in adopting a "not-knowing" position (De Jong & Berg, 2008, p. 13), so SFBT practitioners act as coaches who "lead from one step behind" (p. 13). They maintain their solution-focused language throughout sessions.

SFBT assumptions and tenets

As you are reading, consider key assumptions the SFBT therapist makes. Do you agree? What epistemology underlies these assumptions?

SFBT KEY ASSUMPTIONS

- There are no "a priori" case assumptions. Every client is different.
- Clients already possess the strengths, skills, and competencies to solve their problems.
- The client is the expert on their own life.
- There are always **exceptions**.
- The client defines the treatment goal.
- There is more than one path to a solution.
- Small changes lead to big changes.
- Change occurs all the time; there is no such thing as stability.
- You do not need to know a lot about the problem; therapists should focus on the future.
- There is no such thing as "resistance."
- Clients are doing the best they can.

- SFBT practitioners should use *solution-talk*—not *problem-talk*. (This is discussed in the next two chapters.)

> *(Source material: Bannink, 2007; Bavelas et al., 2013; de Shazer, 1984; Dolan; Duncan et al., 2011; Franklin, 2012; Reiter, 2013; Trepper et al.)*

Basic tenets

The following is a list of SFBT's basic tenets:

a. "It is based on **solution-building** rather than problem-solving.
b. The therapeutic focus should be on the client's desired future rather than on past problems or current conflicts.
c. Clients are encouraged to increase the frequency of current useful behaviors.
d. No problem happens all the time. There are exceptions—that is, times when the problem could have happened but didn't—that can be used by the client and therapist to co-construct solutions.
e. Therapists help clients find alternatives to current undesired patterns of behavior, cognition, and interactions that are within the clients' repertoire or can be co-constructed by therapists and clients as such.
f. Differing from skill building and behavior therapy interventions, the model assumes that solution behaviors already exist for clients.
g. It is asserted that small increments of change lead to large increments of change.
h. Clients' solutions are not necessarily directly related to any identified problem by either the client or the therapist.
i. The conversational skills required of the therapist to invite the client to build solutions are different from those needed to diagnose and treat client problems." (Bavelas et al., 2013, p. 2)

Let's unpack these one at a time.

Tenet 1: "It is based on solution-building rather than problem-solving."

This is the *If it ain't broke, don't fix it* (aka, "If it's not broken, don't fix it") tenet (Dolan, p. 34). Since Freud, many modernist psychotherapeutic models set the tone for understanding that the process of therapy was to get to the "root of the problem" in order to "fix the problem." Those models looked *inside* a person. Yet the modernist folks who created MRI in 1958 (Visser) made a paradigmatic shift because they (1) believed that it may not be necessary to understand the origin of problems (Bannink, 2007) and (2) that the problem was not inside a person but within/between a system (de Shazer, 1982). The problem, they argued, was not the problem—the problem was the failed solution attempt. With Bateson's influence, MRI looked for the "difference that makes a difference" (p. 5) in a system of relationships. This did not carry MRI out of modernist territory (because they held a belief in a single truth and single reality), but it did carry them out of the psychoanalytic tradition and into family therapy. This change helped shift the focus to the present. This is the part of MRI that remains in SFBT: the focus on the here-and-now instead of a so-called root.

In creating SFBT, Berg and de Shazer adopted a view that a therapist need not solve an impossible puzzle. Furthermore, they thought the therapist should reinforce the client's own resources, empowering clients toward their own solutions. This is why SFBT therapists can call themselves "coaches." SFBT highlights what has worked in the past and what is currently working, building upon those as solutions. It is worth reiterating that SFBT therapists do not look for *the* solution but *a* solution. This slight grammatical change should help you remember that SFBT therapists do *not* problem-solve but instead look to solution-building. A solution-building mindset will help the therapist orient toward the future instead of the past, which leads us to the second tenet.

SOLUTION-BUILDING RATHER THAN PROBLEM-SOLVING

Avoid dwelling on the problem. Highlight strengths, resources, and resiliencies. Explore exceptions to the problem. For example, with truancy as the presenting problem, highlight times when the student was not truant or when the issue was less severe.

Tenet 2: "The therapeutic focus should be on the client's desired future rather than on past problems or current conflicts."

In SFBT you will want to avoid rummaging for past traumas or even present conflicts. Allow clients to use their pre-existing strengths and successes and apply them to their current circumstances. Sidestep the temptation to bring about more details about a conflict or problem than necessary. Think about it this way: As an SFBT therapist, you touch on the past like it is a hot stove before you jump to how that applies in the present and the future. If you stay too long, you will get burned. The caveat to this, of course, is that you want to make sure your client feels heard, validated, and that you understand the problem. However, if you stay too long on the problem instead of the client's desired future, you have fallen back into MRI territory, and you will likely end up exploring patterns and communication instead of meaning(s). When a therapist focuses on the client's desired future, they amplify their strengths instead of starting from "square one" of tackling the "root" or "finding out what is *really* going on." As a postmodern model, there is no "really going on" to "discover"—just a punctuation of story (de Shazer, 1982).

Tenet 3: "Clients are encouraged to increase the frequency of current useful behaviors."

The third tenet can be boiled down to: *"If it works, do more of it"* (Reiter, 2014, p. 111). SFBT therapists work as coaches to highlight and reinforce the strengths they see in what the client is doing in the present, inviting clients to increase the frequency of these behaviors. This explains why the model is compliment-heavy and the role of the SFBT therapist is frequently described as a "cheerleader." Notice the tenet uses to the word "useful" instead of "good." As a social constructionist model, SFBT does not make any claims or judgement values on what is good or bad, only more or less useful *for the client.*

Tenet 4: "No problem happens all the time. There are exceptions—that is, times when the problem could have happened but didn't—that can be used by the client and therapist to co-construct solutions."

Clients can come into the therapy room feeling they have exhausted all other options. They may not be able to see the positives in what they have already done, so highlighting exceptions, the fourth tenet, inspires hope that the problem is not a problem all the time. Suddenly, the problem becomes manageable.

The fourth tenet emphasizes how a therapist can know what is more or less useful for a client—by finding times "x" worked well. Berg and de Shazer saw clients as resourceful already, so they worked to point out times when the problem could have occurred but did not occur. From Berg and de Shazer's view, there is always variability in a problem being a problem, as well as to what extent something is a problem.

An SFBT therapist's hard work lies in expanding upon exceptions—times when the problem was not a problem—and building upon those exceptions with the client. Being postmodern, there is not one universal best solution nor exception. There are many different solutions that the client and therapist can try, and it is not up to the therapist to decide the best way (de Shazer et al.). Whatever works in co-constructing solutions!

Tenet 5: "Therapists help clients find alternatives to current undesired patterns of behavior, cognition, and interactions that are within the clients' repertoire or can be co-constructed by therapists and clients as such."

This is the *"If it's not working, do something different"* tenet (Dolan, p. 38). This tenet reinforces that an SFBT therapist supports clients in discovering new possibilities—new patterns of thoughts, behaviors, and interactions. Notice this tenet's use of the word "alternatives" (plural). This is not meant to imply the client needs more skills or coping mechanisms, as someone from a modernist psychotherapeutic (e.g., cognitive-behavioral therapy (CBT)) lens might assume. Again, here is the idea that there are theoretically endless possible solutions. The therapist does not delve into psychoeducation in this case. They lead with curiosity, leaving space for the client to talk about what has worked and what they think might work for them going forward. Dolan used the example of "Seth" who said, "I want to stop eating food that is bad for me." A CBT practitioner might ask, "What are the thoughts you're having before eating the bad food?" to challenge the thought. Whereas the SFBT practitioner replies, "Let's imagine that you succeed in doing exactly that. What will other people in your life (family, friends, co-workers, etc.) notice you doing differently?" (p. 39). In SFBT, the therapist adopts a supportive position, not an instructive, didactic position.

Tenet 6: "Differing from skill building and behavior therapy interventions, the model assumes that solution behaviors already exist for clients."

SFBT therapists assume their clients already have the strengths and abilities to change their situation (Trepper et al.) Like the modernist SMART goals' letter "A," this sixth tenet is about finding attainable steps the client can do. However, a therapist does not have to teach clients how to act differently in a situation, they can simply inquire as to how a good outcome has occurred in the past, exploring more as a coach than an expert providing psychoeducation or teaching skill-building.

The SFBT therapist helps the client use strengths and actions that are already in the client's wheelhouse—not "toolbox" because toolbox implies a set of skills whereas wheelhouse implies one's area of expertise or interest. A toolbox means you are teaching them tools, and a wheelhouse refers to something they have already mastered. SFBT therapists often highlight this as yet another example of a difference between their model and CBT:

> A cognitive-behavioral therapist might respond to a client's description of a good week in a solution-focused manner by exploring what the client did that was helpful in making it a good week. But they would likely also ask about whether the client utilized the CBT skills taught in the previous session.
>
> *(Dolan, p. 19)*

Tenet 7: "It is asserted that small increments of change lead to large increments of change."

The seventh tenet of SFBT is that small changes lead to big changes and sometimes "good enough is good enough." Putting it bluntly, you do not have to hold the client's hand too much. The SFBT therapist trusts in the client's competency and experience go out into the world and continue their upward trajectory. SFBT is simply centered around that *one* presenting problem the client came in for, which is in part what allows this type of therapy to be *brief*. And SFBT practitioners believe that even a baby step along the right path may be all the client needs.

Tenet 8: "Clients' solutions are not necessarily directly related to any identified problem by either the client or the therapist."

Dolan (p. 41) recalled a heartwarming tale of a client whose presenting problem was the passing of her husband and how she felt better after adopting a stray dog. We never know exactly what will help with clients, and SFBT therapists take whatever works—in or out of the therapy room! Recall how, unlike many other models, SFBT does not need to see and analyze all pieces of the puzzle. There is no need to analyze the problem "well enough" to be able to come to the presumed "perfect" solution through even more analysis. The solution might not directly relate to the presenting problem at all, as Dolan said. And the improvement, not necessarily the means, is what the SFBT therapist is looking for.

Tenet 9: "The conversational skills required of the therapist to invite the client to build solutions are different from those needed to diagnose and treat client problems."

The ninth tenet reinforces what you know by now: you do not need to know the "root" of the problem. An SFBT therapist/coach might say: "We don't have to know where the 'underlying anxiety' is coming from. What's helping?" Therefore, since the therapist is not diagnosing or treating, the SFBT therapist is using language differently—as an *activity*—so their conversational, therapeutic expertise will look different from traditional expectations (de Shazer, 1994).

Therapist X: "How many times did you miss school over the past three weeks?"
SFBT Coach: "How many times did you manage to successfully attend the classes this past week? … That's two days more than last week. How did you do it? (Dolan, p. 42)

Part of the SFBT conversational skill is developing the habit of "solution-talk" instead of "problem-talk." These concepts and their connections to the philosopher Wittgenstein are addressed later on. Language and relationship are key.

THE ROLE OF THE SOLUTION FOCUSED BRIEF THERAPIST

The SFBT therapist approaches cases from a non-expert, not-knowing, and—contrary to popular belief—non-manualized approach (de Shazer et al.). The founders would use the language of *"interview"* (Lipckik & de Shazer) instead of "session" to bring the emphasis on the non-pathologizing, collaborative, and non-expert aspects of SFBT. Additionally, it is common for SFBT practitioners to call themselves *"coaches"* instead of "therapists" or "social workers." Although SFBT is complete with questions that *could* compose a manual (i.e., miracle questions, scaling questions, exception questions, coping questions, goal-setting questions, compliments, and solution-focused "homework" assignments), it is not the therapist's job to work step by step as one would with CBT.

As SFBT therapists will continually remind you, a therapist's focus should be on "the process, not the content of the dialogue" (Miller et al., 1991, p. 300). Lipchik (p. 74) offered the example of a family who talks about serious issues (i.e., content) in a light-hearted manner (i.e., process). Therapists, especially newer therapists, can be so distracted by the content and "red herrings" of a conversation that they lose sight of where they are going. There is some content the client will give you that simply does not fall under the "pertinent information" category. Some content seems relevant but can lead you into a dead end. Consider the examples below.

A Less Useful Start:

Therapist X: How are you, and what would you like to talk about today?

Client: Well, I know one thing. I can't have the perfect relationship, job, and living situation all at the same time.

Therapist X: What prompted these feelings? What specifically came up this week?

Client: I just found out my boyfriend is dating my best friend, my roommate knew about it, and my boss is stealing my ideas again.

Therapist X: How did you find out about the affair? ... What exactly happened with your boss? ... Let's dive deeper into that.

In this example, the therapist has "taken the bait," focusing on the content of what the client is sharing instead of the process. The minutia—the tiny details about what happened during the problem—are not important relative to solution-building. What should be fleshed out are the details about the client's resilience, strengths, and resources. This focus on process over content helps clients become "unstuck" (Lipchik), which can be generalized across multiple realms and not just this week's drama.

A More Useful Start:

SFBT Coach: Hi, Val. "So what is better, even a little bit, since we last met?" (de Shazer et al., p. 23)

Client: Nothing is better. My life is falling apart. I just found out my boyfriend is dating my best friend, my roommate knew about it, and my boss is stealing my ideas again.

SFBT Coach: "Wow, you are in a tough situation, and I don't envy your position right now" (Berg & Szabó, p. 128). "How are you managing to cope with this to the degree that you are?" (de Shazer et al., p. 20)

Client: I don't know. Just one foot in front of the other, I suppose.

SFBT Coach: "Good for you!" (Kim, p. 63) … Tell me, "What is one small thing that you could do in the next 24 hours that would help you move, even a little bit, in the direction you want your life to be?" (Dolan, p. 32)

The SFBT therapist always assumes the client is doing the best they can, and that they have tried many solutions on their own. Your job, therefore, is not to "fix" but to highlight their strengths—to allow them to see how they have already succeeded in the past and give them hope they can do it again. This is a more empowering stance on the part of the therapist than a training stance. Some therapists describe this as retaining a focus on the *process* of "*doing* therapy" (de Shazer & Berg, 1992) instead of a focus on giving a client answers.

The therapeutic process itself, taking place in language, is constructive. This is why postmodernists often talk about postmodern therapy being more of an art than a science. The way we speak with one another requires a certain skill, of course, but this is a skill of managing a conversation, not managing a client's life: telling them what to do and not to do. The skill Berg and de Shazer cultivated was using "solution-talk," and framing conversations in positive perspectives, as we discuss in-depth in Chapters 8 and 9.

As an SFBT therapist, you reduce the expert/client dichotomy by reducing a focus on what a therapist is going to "give" to a client and instead thinking about the process of "doing" therapy. Now that we have covered the overview of what an SFBT therapist's role is, I quickly explain the general components that most practitioners take away from the model.

WHAT SFBT PRACTITIONERS DO IN PRACTICE: CONCEPTS AND TECHNIQUES

Unlike other family therapy postmodern family therapy models, SFBT is comfortable with the language of "techniques," coming, no doubt, from MRI's influence of interventions and strategic questioning. However, the techniques are not used in isolation, nor does every one need to be applied as a recipe. The important concepts and techniques are in language.

Miracle question

The miracle question is often used throughout an entire session, not as a single question (see Bavelas et al.). It is intended to get clients thinking about the future and setting goals. It helps the process of changing from problem-talk to solution-talk.

The miracle question usually goes something like, "If you go to bed tonight and a miracle happens while you are asleep, and when you wake up in the morning your problem is solved, how will things be different?" (Lipchik, p. 29). Although the miracle question is arguably the most famous SFBT question, it is by no means necessary. SFBT therapists do *not* have to use the miracle question in their therapy sessions, which would be "checking off the boxes" rather than *doing therapy* (de Shazer & Berg, 1992).

As (de Shazer et al.) explained in their book, *More Than Miracles*, you can do SFBT without ever asking a miracle question. Interestingly, Insoo Kim Berg came up with the miracle question out-of-the-blue when working with a client who kept replying, "I don't know." The miracle question gets clients who are not able to articulate their goals to work backward from an ideal world to small changes that lead to bigger changes (see key assumptions). An SFBT practitioner would ask, "Okay, so suppose a miracle happens and all these problems are over, what would happen instead?" (De Jong) in order to get a goal. Really, the "instead questions" are the turning point, not necessarily the miracle itself (Dolan). If a goal is already identified and framed in solution-talk, there is no need for a miracle question.

An SFBT therapist does not figuratively (or literally, which would be horrendous) wag their finger at a client for not accomplishing a goal. They encourage, not chide. Do not forget that according to this model's assumptions, you do not necessarily need to get to a complete solution—you are solution-building. From an SFBT perspective, sometimes an 8/10 *is* a 10/10 and close enough is good enough. This why SFBT is a *brief* therapy. The actual "miracle" is useful because it takes a problem that seems huge, unsolvable, and overwhelming; and it makes change seem not just possible but also likely. In SFBT, you highlight for the client how their skills, relationships, and traits can come together toward their solution.

Scaling questions

Unlike most scales used to measure something based on normative standards (i.e., a scale that measures and compares the client's functioning with that of the general population along the bell curve), our scales are designed primarily to facilitate treatment. Our scales are used not only to "measure" the client's own perception but also to motivate and encourage, and to elucidate goals, solutions, and anything else that is important to each individual client. ... Scales allow both therapist and client to use the way dialogue works naturally by developing an agreed upon term (i.e., "6") and a concept (i.e., on a scale where "10" stands for the solution and "0" for the starting point, "6" is clearly better than "5") that is obviously multiple and flexible. Since you cannot be absolutely certain what another person meant by his or her use of a word or concept, scaling questions allow both therapist and client to jointly construct a bridge, a way of talking about things that are hard to describe – including progress toward the client's solution.

(de Shazer, 1994, p. 92, as cited
in Korman et al., p. 20)

When you ask a client, "On a scale of 1 to 10, how hopeful are you that you can move up a point from a 5 to 6?," you are not seeking a medicalized, scientific measurement. What you are listening for are the implicit goals, and what you are offering is hope, not merely tracking progress. Scaling questions, then, are intimately tied to the SFBT question, "What's better?"

This is why it is common for SFBT therapists to ask how clients can move up even half a point like from a 5 to a 5.5. As a social constructionist model, SFBT has a laser focus on language. When you introduce scaling questions, make sure you avoid the use of scientific or psychiatric jargon. Scaling questions were intimately tied with de Shazer's practice (de Shazer et al.), and one needs to be cautious with language. Look what de Shazer did to avoid scaling anxiety: "On a scale of 1 to 10, with 10 being that you are as stressed as you can be, and 1 being that you are totally relaxed, where would you say you are today?" (de Shazer, 1991, p. 148, as cited in Lipchik, p. 29). Unlike the system of smiley faces in your local ER, scaling questions need to be non-medicalized—and certainly not diagnostic nor pathologizing. Again, just like the miracle question, this is expanded upon. For example, "How do you know you are at a 6? What tells you that? How do you know you're not at a 4? If Jessica were here today, what number would she say you are? How would she have come up with that number?" and so forth. I think many people ask scaling questions but forget to expand upon them. Counterintuitively, you will want to elicit more details about the solution than the problem.

Exception questions

SFBT therapists presuppose (1) change is possible and (2) that there is a time when the problem is not a problem. Even in the present, there are least a few moments to minutes when the problem is not happening. Exception questions bring about information about the past, but these questions are not meant to delve into the client's past as in searching for a root cause such as in childhood attachment. SFBT therapists ask questions that elicit past successes to create successes in the present and the future. Therefore, you will look for "how" over "why." This allows the SFBT therapist to maintain an overall future-focus even when temporarily stepping into the past. One only looks into the past to find and expand upon "solution-building procedures" instead of "problem-solving procedures" (De Jong & Berg, 2002, p. 16). As De Jong and Berg told readers, "[Peter's colleague] ended her first interview (i.e., session) with what she was already doing to make her miracle happen and suggesting that she do some of the additional things that might make miracle-type days more likely to occur" (p. 16). The focus is on the *doing* not some *root*.

Coping questions

If you ask a client where they are on the scale of hopefulness, and they say a 0, representing not hopeful at all, then you can ask: "What have you done to prevent things from getting worse?" (Lipchik, p. 30). Coping questions can be helpful when clients are reticent to give themselves credit for the work they have already done. Essentially, coping questions ask something along the lines of, "How have you been able to deal with all that?" The question holds within itself an implication of "You're doing great." And it allows the client and therapist to further build upon the exceptions and the client's unique strengths.

Compliments

SFBT therapists often utilize compliments to punctuate and validate what clients are already doing that is useful. You can compliment the client as a person or their efforts. The punctuation is key, so sometimes just saying, "Wow!" can get the job done. It is important to watch your language here because you can give a compliment in two different ways: directly and indirectly (Dolan). Language comes into play once again as a critical component of this postmodern model. The first way you can compliment is by giving a client a direct compliment and the second is by eliciting a self-compliment from the client. "That's great!" is a compliment that comes from the therapist. And, "How did you do that?" is an implied compliment that allows the client to compliment themselves by virtue of answering the question (de Shazer et al.) Compliments allow for positives reframes (Lipchik).

Goal-setting

> The founders and their colleagues soon discovered that they could not simply ask the client, "What is your goal?" When they did that, the client would respond "to stop drinking," or "to stop fighting with my teenage son," or "to be less depressed." These client responses were more like problem statements rather than goals. They began experimenting with questions like, "What are you going to do instead of the drinking?", "When you are not drinking, what will be there instead," and, "What will others notice you doing when you are not drinking anymore?"
>
> *(De Jong, p. 3)*

Questions are the "primary communication tool" in SFBT, and how you ask those questions matters (de Shazer et al., p. 11). SFBT therapists assume clients have often tried out solutions to these same problems before, so with an open-ended question like, "What is your goal?" you may fall into problem-talk. *Instead questions* shift into solution-talk; moving from what clients do *not* want to what they *do* want (Dolan). This helps clients get a better picture of the main features of their desired future.

SFBT therapists use language to create new possible futures. By asking clients about their desired future and working backward, you co-create new goals and possible solutions. These solutions do not have to be fancy. The appeal is in their simplicity.

> … the therapist and client are constructing a therapeutic reality based on continuing transformation or change (as evidenced by any exceptions), rather than on initiating change. When exceptions are identified, the task will usually include

the idea that the client should do more of what they are already doing rather than suggesting that they do something new.

(de Shazer, 1988, p. 5, as cited in
Korman et al., 2020, p. 11)

A solution to increase the frequency of what is working often feels more manageable than a suggestion to do something entirely different—although that is an option too.

Solution-focused homework assignments

This section is worth opening with a direct quote from one of the foremost SFBT authorities. If you have a highlighter, highlight this quote.

> Solution focused therapy practitioners typically refrain from asking clients to do assigned "homework" which is common in many other psychotherapy approaches. However, they sometimes offer clients an optional "experiment" like, "Between now and the next time we meet, I invite you to—whenever you happen to think about it or feel like it—take a moment to pay attention to anything that you or anyone else is doing that somehow helps you move in the direction of your goal.
>
> *(Dolan, p. 12)*

SFBT is known in the psychotherapeutic community for assigning homework to clients. However, it is important to keep in mind that the founders did not conceptualize homework in the same way as one might in CBT or a general workbook. See de Shazer's explanation of an *experiment* as "a nudge":

> Once SFBT therapists have created a positive frame via compliments and then discovered some previous solutions and exceptions to the problem, they gently nudge the client to do more of what has previously worked or to try changes brought up by the client—frequently called 'an experiment' (i.e., homework). It is rare for an SFBT therapist to make a suggestion or assignment that is not based on the client's previous solutions or exceptions. It is always best if change ideas and assignments emanate from the client.
>
> *(de Shazer et al., p. 12)*

It is helpful to separate SFBT's idea of what homework is from a preconceived idea of what homework is in other models. These *experiments* more closely align with MRI directives than CBT skill-building. Differentiating itself from the expert-stanced MRI, however, SFBT therapists support clients in conducting experiments to solve their own problems, usually "leading from one step behind" (Kim, p. 7) in a non-expert position (Lipchik) instead of giving expert directives. Thus experiments are usually offered in tentative language, and the founders worked from a belief that the client should come up with their own experiment, likely focusing on what had already worked and doing more of it (de Shazer et al.).

SUMMARY

Influenced by Bateson, Erickson, and the MRI team, Berg and de Shazer co-created SFBT in the 1980s (de Shazer, 1982). SFBT is an evidence-based model. SFBT was created inductively, meaning it derived from empirical observation of what was working with clients prior to having a set theory. As it developed, SFBT became postmodern, aligning itself with social constructionist ideas (Bannink; Kim). In addition to understanding the key assumptions and basic tenets of SFBT, implementing therapeutic micro-skills such as building rapport is important for positive outcomes (Lipchik & de Shazer).

SFBT therapists do not solve problems (Kim; Dolan). The role of the SFBT therapist/coach/practitioner is to build upon solutions instead (De Jong & Berg). A coach engages personably with clients in solution-oriented interviews/sessions (Lipchik & de Shazer). Language is the epicenter of this model, and de Shazer and Berg highlighted language as a joint process—an *activity* (1992). SFBT practitioners avoid focusing solely on the content of dialogues (Miller et al.) and frankly ask unusual questions for those unaccustomed to it.

Popular practices include miracle questions, exception questions, coping questions, scaling questions, compliments, and "experiments" as homework (de Shazer et al.). Although these are certainly part of what makes SFBT, these are not the only pillars defining the model, and attempts to manualize them should be avoided. SFBT concepts are not boxes to tick off because SFBT is more than just a series of techniques (de Shazer et al.; Lipchik). Although an "empirical social constructionist model" is a little oxymoronic (because empiricism is modern while social constructionism is postmodern), this little paradox of a model has mass appeal.

REFLECTIVE QUESTIONS

1. How does SFBT differ from CBT?
2. How is the therapeutic process of SFBT different from giving advice?
3. How do SMART goals differ from SFBT's goal-setting approach?
4. What is the role of the miracle question?
5. What is the role of exception questions?

Keywords

Brief

Solution-Oriented

Future-Focused

Inductive

Evidence-Based

Exceptions

Solution-Building

Interview

Coach

Doing Therapy

Miracle Questions

Scaling Questions

Exception Questions

Coping Questions

Goal-Setting Questions

Compliments

Experiments

Solution Focused Brief Therapy Post-Test (Inspired by Lipchik, 2011)

1. Why is it important to acknowledge MRI's influence?
   a. Bateson, Erickson, Jackson, Haley, Weakland, and Watzlawick are not only important figures in family therapy's history, paving the way for the family therapy practices of today, but also critical to understanding Insoo Kim Berg and Steve de Shazer's relational focus and position toward techniques. Since the BFTC, techniques have been embraced in SFBT. Yet is worth noting that C-DP and narrative therapy are more cautious about using "techniques." Anderson outright rejected the term, and White explained how externalization is better understood as conversations than a technique. Acknowledging MRI's influence is acknowledging the importance of modernist thought still underlying this model. There is an argument that SFBT is not postmodern or not *as* postmodern as the other two models because of this lineage.

2. How are emotions addressed in SFBT?
   a. This is a good question, and the next two chapters will shed light on how de Shazer and Berg thought about emotions in SFBT. For now, I answer that emotions are acknowledged, and clients' feelings are validated. However, SFBT practitioners ignore the illusion of a "root" emotion or "root" cause.

3. "How do I know I am being solution-focused?" (p. 17)
   a. If you are being solution-focused instead of deficit-focused, you have achieved the first step: orienting toward solutions. Next, check to make sure you are being future-focused instead of attending to current or past patterns. You will likely know you are doing this because most practitioners are not used to maintaining future-focused language. Most psychotherapists are trained to get as much detail about the problem as possible. But in SFBT, one might not address the problem at all—only what improvement would be necessary for the clients to be more satisfied or content. After these basics, incorporate SFBT's key assumptions and basic tenets and practice, practice, practice using language differently.

4. "What do I respond to and what do I ignore?" (p. 17)
   a. You will respond to clients' strengths, resiliencies, skills, and successes. Ignore the content or the supposed origin. "Why" questions do not get much attention in SFBT. "How" and "what" questions certainly get more limelight (e.g., "How were you able to do that?" or

"What will others notice when …"). Remember, you are looking for exceptions and how clients have already had bits of their ideal—their "miracle." Here you work on solution-building—building upon what has already worked and likely doing more of it.

5. "Can I do SFT with long-term clients?" (p. 17)

   a. Based on MRI's 10-session approximation and supported by their own research into brief therapy's success, as explained above, SFBT practice had less than 20 sessions. This is what de Shazer had to say on the topic: "For some years it's been that brief therapy means, among other things, 'as few sessions as possible and not one more than necessary'" (as quoted in Hoyt, 1996, p. 61). Some people do it for years and others for single-session therapy. Insoo Kim Berg might have asked, "If you can come to a solution in one session, why would you extend the therapy beyond that? Longer SFBT sessions bring up ethical questions. For whom are these sessions scheduled? After all, *brief* is in the name. If research shows effective SFBT therapy in four (Hoyt) or six sessions (De Jong), and you are forbidden from exploring any "root" cause or origin, what are you doing in your longer sessions? I believe that whatever you choose, you must ethically support your decision(s) with primary sources, relevant codes of ethics, site policies, and state laws.

6. I have tried SFBT, but it is not working. I keep trying to stay away from the problem, and my client keeps falling back into the problem. What am I doing wrong?

   a. It may be the case that this therapist skipped the critical step of defining the goal, not only in meaning but also in behaviors, that is, what will it *look like* when they have reached their goal? This way, when it happens, or when a bit of it happens, the clients can notice it. It could also be the case that the client did not feel the therapist was listening. The therapist should acknowledge what the client says is the problem and only after that move toward defining an attainable goal. Furthermore, have you ever noticed that sometimes the more you try to do a model, the less successful you feel you are as a therapist? This is often the case for newer practitioners. My advice here is not to discard the model but to practice until it becomes second nature. And if you are using a model that is antithetical to your epistemology, it will not become second nature. Thus it is important to discover your personal epistemology to see if it is compatible with what you are trying to practice. Afterward, you can work on refining what you feel compelled to do with the parameters of the model.

7. Can I combine/integrate SFBT with other models?

   a. The answer depends on who you ask. Although there is plenty of research to support integration, de Shazer himself said no (2016) and that it would be akin seeing out of one eye instead of two. Instead, he recommended that you learn multiple models and be able to switch from one model to another. This way you are seeing things clearly every time. Think of it as switching out one pair of glasses for another rather than trying bifocals (see de Shazer, 2016).

8. These questions seem inauthentic. How do I make it my own?

   a. It may be this model is not a good "fit" (2016) for you. Or it may be that you are not practiced in asking these questions and using language in this way, which is quite understandable. I would suggest remembering to contextualize the questions. Context—not content—is everything. Continue reading the next two chapters and see whether this improves your comfort level with SFBT practices. If you find you are less inclined to learn more about it, you may have your answer. But I caution you against claiming you practice SFBT while not understanding and applying its theory/philosophy/epistemology. Eve Lipchik described theory as "part of everything we do" (p. 34). If you ignore the theory and only apply techniques, I would argue you are not doing SFBT.

9. What are fundamental SFBT components?

   a. This is an interesting question to consider. What happens if you take the *solution-focus* out of SFBT? It becomes, more or less, MRI. What happens if you take the *brief* out of SFBT? It becomes solution-oriented therapy. What happens if you take the *therapy* out of SFBT? It becomes coaching. Perhaps, like C-DP or narrative therapy, the name of the model itself reveals the most fundamental components.

NOTE

1 NB: These BFTC sessions are not the same as Tom Andersen's reflecting team practice nor Michael White's outsider witness practice which were each done transparently and conversationally with the clients.

STEVE DE SHAZER AND INSOO KIM BERG: PRIMARY SOURCES

Berg, I. K. (1994). *Family based services: A solution-focused approach.* W. W. Norton & Company.

Berg, I. K., & Szabó, P. (2005). *Brief coaching for lasting solutions.* W. W. Norton.

De Jong, P., & Berg, I. K. (2002). *Interviewing for solutions* (2nd ed.). Wadsworth.

De Jong, P., & Berg, I. K. (2008). *Instructor's resource manual for "Interviewing for solutions"* (4th ed.). Cengage.

de Shazer, S. (1982). *Patterns of brief family therapy.* The Guilford Press.

de Shazer, S. (1984). The death of resistance. *Family Process, 23,* 79–93.

de Shazer, S. (1991). *Putting difference to work.* W. W. Norton & Company.

de Shazer, S. (1994). *Words were originally magic.* W. W. Norton & Co.

de Shazer, S. (1997). Some thoughts on language use in therapy. *Contemporary Family Therapy, 19*(1), 133–141.

de Shazer, S. (2016). Fit. *Journal of Systemic Therapies, 35*(1), 55–59.

de Shazer, S., & Berg, I. K. (1992). Doing therapy: A post-structural re-vision. *Journal of Marital and Family Therapy, 18*(1), 71–81.

de Shazer, S., Dolan, Y., Korman, H., Trepper, T., McCollum, T., & Berg, I. K. (2021). *More than miracles: The state of the art of solution focused brief therapy* (2nd dig. ed.). Routledge.

Lipchik, E., & de Shazer, S. (2017). The purposeful interview. *Journal of Systemic Therapies, 36*(2), 54–66.

Renowned Sources

Anderson, H. (2015). Postmodern/poststructural/social construction therapies: Collaborative, narrative, and solution-focused. In T. L. Sexton & J. Lebow (Ed.), *Handbook of family therapy: The science and practice of working with families and couples* (1st dig. ed., pp. 182–204). Routledge.

Bavelas, J., De Jong, P., Franklin, C., Froerer, A., Gingerich, W., Kim, J., Korman, H., Langer, S., Lee, M. Y., McCollum, E. E., Jordan, S. S., & Trepper, T. S. (2013). Solution focused therapy treatment manual for working with individuals (2nd version). *Solution Focused Brief Therapy Association*.

De Jong, P. (2019). A brief, informal history of SFBT as told by Steve de Shazer and Insoo Kim Berg. *Journal of Solution Focused Practices*, 3(1), 1–5.

Dolan, Y. (2024). *Solution focused therapy: The basics* (1st dig. ed.). Routledge.

Duncan, B. L., Miller, S. D., & Sparks, J. A. (2011). *The heroic client: A revolutionary way to improve effectiveness through client-directed, outcome-informed therapy*. John Wiley & Sons.

Franklin, C. (Ed.). (2012). *Solution-focused brief therapy: A handbook of evidence-based practice*. Oxford University Press.

Froerer, A., von Cziffra-Bergs, J., Kim, J., & Connie, E. (2018). *Solution-focused brief therapy with clients managing trauma*. Oxford University Press.

Kim, J. S. (Ed.) (2013). *Solution focused brief therapy: A multicultural approach*. Sage.

Kim, J., Jordan, S. S., Franklin, C., & Froerer, A. (2019). Is solution-focused brief therapy evidence-based? An update 10 years later. Families in society. *Sage Journals*, 100(2), 127–138.

Korman, H., De Jong, P., & Jordan, S. S. (2020). Steve de Shazer's theory of development. *Journal of Solution Focused Practices*, 4(2), 47–70.

Lipchik, E. (2011). *Beyond technique in solution focused brief therapy: Working with emotions and the therapeutic relationship* (dig. ed.). Guilford.

Miller, S. D., Hubble, M. A., & Duncan, B. L. (1991). *Handbook of solution focused brief therapy*. Jossey-Bass.

Trepper, T. S., McCollum, E. E., De Jong, P., Korman, H., Gingerich, W., & Franklin, C. (2013). Solution-focused therapy treatment manual for working with individuals. In J. S. Kim (Ed.), *Solution-focused brief therapy: A multicultural approach* (pp. 14–31). Sage.

Additional References

Bannink, F. P. (2007). Solution focused brief therapy. *Journal of Contemporary Psychotherapy*, 37, 87–94.

Berquez, A., & Jeffery, M. (2024). *Solution focused brief therapy with children and young people who stammer and their parents: A practical guide from the Michael Palin Centre*. Routledge.

Chenail, R. J., Reiter, M. D., Torres-Gregory, M., & Ilic, D. (2020). Postmodern family therapy. *The Handbook of Systemic Family Therapy*, 1, 417–442.

Durrant, M. (2007). Remembering Insoo Kim Berg. *Journal of Systemic Therapies*, 26(2), 1–12.

Hoyt, M. F. (Ed.). (1996). *Constructive therapies* (Vol. 2). Guilford Press.

Internet Encyclopedia of Philosophy. (2024). *Deductive and inductive arguments*. https://iep.utm.edu/deductive-inductive-arguments/

Lee, M. Y. (2011). Solution-focused theory. In F. J. Turner (Ed.), *Social work treatment: Interlocking theoretical approaches* (pp. 513–609). Oxford University Press.

Macdonald, A. J. (2011). *Solution focused therapy: Theory, research, and practice*. Sage.

Macdonald, A. J. (2016). Encounters with Steve de Shazer and Insoo Kim Berg: Inside stories of solution focused brief therapy. *Journal of Solution Focused Practices*, 2(1), 67–69.

Pichot, T. (2014). *de Shazer, Steve*. Encyclopedia of social work. https://doi.org/10.1093/acrefore/9780199975839.013.1120

Reiter, M. D. (2013). *Case conceptualization in family therapy*. Pearson.

Reiter, M. D. (2017). *Family therapy: An introduction to process, practice, and theory*. Routledge.

Soiferman, K. (2010). *Compare and contrast inductive and deductive research approaches* [Online submission]. ERIC.

Visser, C. F. (2013). The origin of the solution-focused approach. *International Journal of Solution-Focused Practices*, 1(1), 10–17.

CHAPTER 8

Ludwig Wittgenstein

....

Remember, as you read through these chapters, you can always return to the Introduction to refresh your memory on the terms you learned, such as metaphysics, positivism, and ontology.

QUESTIONS TO THINK ABOUT

1. What are the seminal texts associated with Ludwig Wittgenstein?
2. In what ways did Wittgenstein's philosophy change over time?
3. What is the relationship between games and language games?
4. What does Wittgenstein's "beetle in the box" indicate?
5. What is Wittgenstein's private language argument?

Austrian philosopher Ludwig Wittgenstein (pronounced "Lud-vig Vit-guhn shtahyn") is known for his radical ideas. Some think of him as a philosopher's philosopher; others think of him as an anti-philosopher. "Early-Wittgenstein" thought his work, the *Tractatus*, resolved all philosophical muddles forever such that philosophy was no longer needed (Grayling, 2001). Whereas "late-Wittgenstein" would directly contradict this and go against many of his earlier beliefs (Monk, 2019).

As Wittgenstein himself lamented, most people did not understand him, and we certainly cannot ask for clarification from beyond the grave. Since there is no absolute consensus on Wittgenstein's philosophy, I gathered support from multiple, esteemed experts on Wittgenstein and his works. In addition to my own comments upon Wittgenstein's work, I pulled from authorities Ray Monk, Cora Diamond, David Cockburn, Lars Hertzberg, James Klagge, A. C. Grayling, and Miles Hollingworth. By my estimation, Ray Monk (2019) is among the most eminent Wittgensteinian scholars, sharing the spotlight with celebrated philosopher and scholar Cora Diamond (2017). I recommend

DOI: 10.4324/9781003439349-12

readers looking for a deep Wittgensteinian understanding to start here. I also included works by well-regarded Wittgensteinian scholars David Cockburn (2022, 2023) and Lars Hertzberg (2022), and James C. Klagge (2016) who offer substantial contributions in their own right. I considered including the notorious Saul Kripke, eventually deciding against it to avoid confusion between Wittgenstein and what has been termed "Kripkenstein." My choices are not merely based on personal opinion; the scholars I included are all recognized authorities by the British Wittgenstein Society. I have additionally relied on biographers Miles Hollingworth (2018) and A. C. Grayling (2001) for their well-known introductions to Wittgenstein. I recommend these latter authors for readers searching for lighter reading on the philosopher's life. I included supplementary sources in this chapter as further support for my comments.

Even the above-mentioned scholars disagree with one another about Wittgenstein's content and intention. However, they agree that Wittgenstein was anti-theoretical. His philosophy was clearly in contrast to the so-called armchair philosophers who theorized about abstract concepts and asked Platonic (i.e., referring to Plato) questions like, "What is Beauty? (capital 'B')" rather than, as Wittgenstein would have suggested, looking at what things were "beautiful" (lowercase "b").

This chapter offers a way to read Wittgenstein, but it is not the only way to read Wittgenstein. Nevertheless, I believe my comments on Wittgenstein match more closely than not with remarks from family therapy founders Steve de Shazer, Michael White, and Harlene Anderson. Chapter 9 addresses which Wittgensteinian thoughts resonated with family therapy pioneers Steve de Shazer and Insoo Kim Berg and how solution focused brief therapy's (SFBT) technique of solution-talk connects with Wittgenstein's philosophy.

WHO WAS LUDWIG WITTGENSTEIN?

As Smith (2021) and Grayling (2001) said, Austrian philosopher Ludwig Wittgenstein was one of the greatest and most eccentric philosophers of the 20th century, living a fascinating life from 1889 to 1951. As may be of interest to my Bowenian readers and others interested in sibling position, Monk and Hollingworth shared that Ludwig Wittgenstein was the youngest of a large family of eight children, and three of his four older brothers died by suicide: Johannes (Hans), Rudolf (Rudi), and Kurt. Scholars and biographers speculate about the role their authoritarian father Karl Wittgenstein may have played in his five sons' depression and suicidality throughout their lives (Klagge). Rumors also exist about whether one or more of his brothers, like Ludwig, was gay and filled with self-loathing for the "perversion"—which, poignantly, their contemporary Sigmund Freud would go on to "treat" as part of his practice in the Wittgenstein's hometown of Vienna in the 1920s, even seeing Wittgenstein's sister as a patient for psychoanalysis (Eilenberger, 2020; Peters, 2019). From Peters' (2019, 2022) and Smith's descriptions, it seems there may have been an additional level of Jewish self-hatred in "non-religious" (Klagge), "God-obsessed" (Peters) Ludwig Wittgenstein's unique intersectionality of Jewish heritage, Catholic baptism, regular Christian practices, and religious mysticism (2022, p. 1954).

According to Monk, Hollingworth, and Grayling, Wittgenstein's family gained wealth and stature not only from intergenerational wealth but also from his father's practically monopolized iron and steel business in Vienna. His family's affluence afforded Wittgenstein opportunities to be exposed to intellectual and cultural elites, which spurred his interests in music, logic, engineering, language, mathematics, and philosophy; he had recurrent occasions to keep company with famous composers like Gustav Mahler and Richard Strauss and famous artists like Gustav Klimt (Hollingworth). Klimt, indeed, best known for his gold-leaf masterpiece, "The Kiss," painted a portrait of Wittgenstein's sister Margaret "Gretl" Stonborough-Wittgenstein in 1905 (Klagge). This is currently on display in the Neue Pinakothek art museum. The Wittgenstein family was clearly very well connected in Austria.

As Diamond and Grayling each explained, Wittgenstein pursued engineering in Manchester before meeting with the famous philosopher and mathematician Bertrand Russell, who convinced the branded genius to become a disciple and philosopher instead of an aeronautical engineer. Wittgenstein arrived at Cambridge in 1912 to study under Russell, initially interested in Russell's philosophy of logic and mathematics (Diamond). These two thinkers had immense impacts on each other's fame and philosophical development (Eilenberger; Klagge).

When World War I broke out, Wittgenstein became an Austro-Hungarian army soldier and eventually a prisoner of war in northern Italy (Monk). During the war, Wittgenstein discovered and read a book by Leo Tolstoy called *Gospel in Brief,* which he found deeply moving—although he notably did not like it as much as his favorite novel, Fyodor Dostoyevsky's *The Brothers Karamazov* (Monk; Peters, 2022). Wittgenstein seemingly resonated with these Russian authors' way of showing narrative accounts of ethics and morality, which may be contrasted to a principled, explanatory account like in philosopher Immanuel Kant's work entitled *The Groundwork of the Metaphysics of Morals.* Aligning with the literary characters Alyosha and Father Zosima in *The Brothers Karamazov,* Wittgenstein drastically changed his lavish lifestyle after the war. Wittgenstein gave away his fortune to become an elementary school teacher, gardener, and later an architect for his sister before going back to Cambridge in 1929 to continue his work as a philosopher at the behest of his friend Ramsey (Eilenberger; Grayling; Hollingworth). When he returned to Cambridge with Ramsey, his philosophy had metamorphosed.

Early-Wittgenstein had sought to break down language into its essential arrangements of constituents, analyze its logical, propositional form, and see language as a picture of the world like the sentence, "The cat is on the mat," discarding philosophical language as not representational of reality, that is, non-pictorial (Cockburn, 2022; Diamond; Klagge) and thus not something people could sensibly talk about such as the question, "Is God benevolent?" Early-Wittgenstein applied Russell's teachings of logical and mathematical proofs (Grayling) to philosophy. He believed his contemporaries and those philosophers who preceded him all the way up to Socrates were misunderstanding the mechanics of language and asking the wrong questions, trying to unravel unanswerable metaphysical (i.e., referring to *that which lies beyond nature*) and ontological (i.e., referring to *being*) questions. Regardless of his documented interest in God and religion, Wittgenstein thought we did not have the language to be able to speak intelligibly about God or any transcendental philosophy (e.g., ethics or aesthetics); therefore, he thought any attempt to speak about what is *beyond* the world would be a waste of time, and our pictorial language was simply not equipped for it (Grayling;

Monk). Wittgenstein made it clear there was no way we could ever be "outside" of language, outside of our world (Wittgenstein, 1922). He thought philosophical language did not reflect a knowable reality, and so could not be answered; thus, misunderstanding the mathematical-like structure of language is the reason so many great thinkers ended up in muddles (Diamond). Therefore, one could be religious, but to talk about religion would be senseless.

Directly contradicting his early work, late-Wittgenstein's philosophy challenged his own picture-theory of language wherein words are pictures of the world. Wittgenstein was forever changed by a conversation with his Italian friend Piero Sraffa who asked him what the propositional form of an Italian chin flick gesture was, performing it in front of him, which challenged early-Wittgenstein's ways of thinking about language as a system made up of propositions like mathematics and engineering (Klagge). He admitted he had been "seduced into thinking that something quite remarkable was achieved by propositions"; meanwhile, propositions actually trick us into "beginning to think we need an explanation: *'How does this work?'*" (Diamond, 35:33). Wittgenstein then contended that we should avoid this trap: "We need to be able to see—as philosophically relevant—*the familiar, ordinary aspects of things*" (38:45). We need to see that language is inherently social, governed by rules that work in one situation and not in another. So, as Monk explained, late-Wittgenstein discarded his "picture theory" of language and encouraged his students and colleagues to see language in its social, relational context that cannot be isolated and analyzed as something separate. Instead of looking for the explanation of how language works, he said we already know how language operates because we use it every day (Hertzberg), so no atomistic analysis is needed.

> From 1929 until his death in 1951, Wittgenstein worked out a new way of doing philosophy that has no precedent in the history of the subject. It is a way of approaching philosophy that tries to remain faithful to the insight that philosophy *cannot* be a science, or anything like a science. It is not a body of doctrine but an activity, the activity of clearing up the confusions caused by the bewitchments cast by language.
>
> *(Monk, p. vii)*

Late-Wittgensteinian thought is what is best known in philosophy, psychology, linguistics, and other domains and has strongly resonated with pioneers across disciplines. Wittgenstein passed away in 1951. Although his works preceded the postmodern movement, which gained popular culture traction in the 1950s–1960s, his philosophy has been incredibly influential on postmodern models, including SFBT, narrative therapy, and collaborative-dialogic practice.

WHAT DID WITTGENSTEIN WRITE?

Wittgenstein wrote two popularized books: *Tractatus Logico-Philosophicus* and *Philosophical Investigations*. When he wrote the *Tractatus*, Wittgenstein proclaimed that this book was the end of philosophy and genuinely thought he had solved the headaches of philosophical debates (Hollingworth). His later work challenged his earlier ideas, which he addressed in the *Philosophical Investigations*. He confessed that his thinking had changed over the 20–30 years from the time he wrote the *Tractatus* to the time he wrote *Philosophical Investigations*. Even in *Philosophical Investigations*, he explained that the *Investigations* could be seen as a correction to some of his earlier ideas but likely contained errors (Wittgenstein, 2009).

RELEVANT WITTGENSTEINIAN CONCEPTS

The most recognized Wittgensteinian concept is something called *language games*, and it is the central theme of his later book *Philosophical Investigations* (Monk). As a brief overview, this concept brings our attention to the importance of context. Wittgenstein's central point was that our language is tied to our everyday activities, so we should not create a detachment between life and language (Hertzberg, 2022). Rather than imagining language as something one employs to represent a factual world, one should see the complexities of how we were taught language *in* the world. Aside from proper names and a few other instances, our words do not directly refer to a clear entity. We truly learn what words mean through contextualized examples, not abstract definitions. Wittgenstein pointed out that when we are taught language as babies or as adults learning a new language, teachers will use examples until they are sure the person understands. This is then demonstrated by the person's ability to correctly use the word in its proper context, not to offer the perfect definition.

Late-Wittgenstein rejected a one-to-one correspondence between words and the objects they denote, and Wittgenstein's exploration of language games illuminated the fluid nature of language, dispelling the notion that words are pictures of the world. Language, from this vantage point, is not one unified thing, but rather functions in different ways through an intricate web of linguistic rules and social conventions in different spheres of life. One way to put it is that late-Wittgenstein focused on the many languages we use (as in contextually—not literally such as English, Spanish, French, etc.) instead of focusing on trying to find an isolated theory to explain Language (capital "L").

BRIEF SUMMARY AND ANALYSIS OF LATE-WITTGENSTEIN'S FAMOUS WORK

Wittgenstein is one of the most difficult philosophers to read. This is not for the usual reason of being dense and using highly academic, philosophical language, but because of the seeming disorganization of his second book. His first book mirrored logical or mathematical proofs as one point would build off another. In his second book, his thoughts are scattered.

Philosophical investigations (1953)

Philosophical Investigations was published in an incomplete state after Wittgenstein's death in 1951. It is certainly unique in its structure in that it is a collection of numbered paragraphs. These sections do not necessarily flow together and can appear quite random and sporadic. In the *Investigations*, he used metaphors and similes rather than relying on propositions.

Wittgenstein opened the first section by quoting philosopher and theologian Augustine:

When grown-ups named some object and at the same time turned towards it, I perceived this, and I grasped that *the thing was signified by the sound they uttered*, since they meant to point it out. This, however, I gathered from their gestures, the natural language of all peoples, the language that by means of facial expression and the play of eyes, of the movements of the limbs and the tone of voice, indicates the affections of the soul when it desires, or clings to, or rejects, or recoils from, something. In this way, little by little, I learnt to understand what things the words, which I heard uttered in their respective places in various sentences, signified. And once I got my tongue around these signs, I used them to express my wishes.

(Wittgenstein, 2009, p. 5, italics added for emphasis)

He immediately followed this quote with:

These words, it seems to me, give us a particular picture of the *essence of human language*. It is this: the *words in language name objects*——sentences are combinations of such names. ——In this picture of language, we find the roots of the following idea: *Every word has a meaning. This meaning is correlated with the word*. It is the object for which the word stands. Augustine *does not* mention any difference between *kinds* of words. Someone who describes the learning of language in this way is, I believe, thinking primarily of nouns like "table," "chair," and "bread," and of people's names, and only secondarily of the names of certain actions and properties; and of the remaining kinds of words as something that will "take care of itself."

(p. 5, italics added for emphasis)

As I mentioned, Wittgenstein, originally a mathematician, engineer, and logician, had by this time stopped believing the dominant theory that there was an "essence of human language"—unlike most philosophers and academics of his time (Monk). His predecessors and contemporaries had been looking to discover "the essence" of things, like beauty, virtue, or language, since the established origins of Western philosophy. Wittgenstein can, therefore, be interpreted as refuting Augustine's stance that the so-called essence would be the "*object* for which the word stands" since, as Wittgenstein pointed out, this does not account for *all* kinds of words, only some words like nouns.

Next, Wittgenstein offered a thought experiment of someone requesting "five red apples" at a market.

I send someone shopping. I give him a slip of paper marked "five red apples." He takes the slip to the shopkeeper, who opens the drawer marked "apples;" then the shopkeeper looks up the word "red" in a chart and finds a color sample next to it; then he says the series of elementary number-words——I assume that he knows them by heart up to the word "five," and for each number-word he takes an apple of the same color as the sample out of the drawer. ——It is in this and similar ways that one operates with words.

(2009, pp. 5–6)

I offer an interpretation which seems to align with common sense (Monk). Realistically, adults who are fluent in English *do not* need a drawer labeled "apples" to figure out what is meant to be communicated by the word "apple," nor do they need a chart labeled "red" to know what is meant to be communicated by the word "red." Therefore, when Wittgenstein said, "It is in this and similar ways that one operates with words," I believe he is either being sarcastic or referencing a different audience for one of his Cambridge lectures: "It is in this and similar ways we are used to thinking about words" becomes, "It is in this and similar ways *an academic* operates with words." This makes his words a criticism of other intellectuals of his time—even of his past self-regarding his "picture theory." Wittgenstein is wondering why very smart people in top academic environments like Cambridge are adopting an overly simplified view of language which, ironically, complicates language by separating it from our experience. The imagined other replied, "——But what is the *meaning* of the word 'five'?" To which Wittgenstein responded, "——No such thing was in question here, only how the word 'five' is used" (p. 6).

As you will see resonated with de Shazer, Wittgenstein's *Investigations* brought abstract philosophical thoughts about language down to practical use. He prompted others to think of what real people actually *do* with words. Even if the shopkeeper did count up to five out loud, there would not be a label that directly correlates. In other words, in a conceptual way (not a written symbol), what does "*a* five" look like? Wittgenstein's point appears to be that people are trained to think about language as though the shopkeeper follows through with the request through the structure of the meaning the object five + the meaning of object red + the meaning of an object apple. But really, when the shopkeeper gathers the apples for the transaction, he already knows what to gather from experience. He does not look for a label to represent each word. Think about "5." Clearly, not all words are "the object for which the word stands."

Furthermore, Wittgenstein argued against language as representational even when we think of a child learning words from flashcards with a word on one side and a picture on the other because, although "a child uses primitive forms of language when they learn to talk, the teaching of language is not *explaining* [meaning], but *training* [in use]" (p. 7). Children enter into language with a pre-existing social context, so they are trained in language; however, intellectuals of his time (and some of ours) persisted in attempts to distill language down to an additive formula of words' essences.

Wittgenstein introduced a second thought experiment. Imagine two builders working where one calls out, "Slab!" which is a stand-in command for, "Bring me a slab." Here the two can be used interchangeably—not because of an absolute shared meaning but because of our awareness of its *use*. This is quite different from "slab" on the one hand always representing a noun or on the other hand always meaning "bring me a slab" (p. 12). How we use words varies depending on context like the social situation and we understand each other perfectly well. Our common sense is showing us we already have a sense of this through our training by living in the world. There is no absolute meaning because context shifts. There is no direct correspondence of a word to an object or an object to reality. This situation where "Slab!" is understood to mean, "Bring me a slab," is an example of the builder's "language game."

Language games

Walking the walk and adhering to his own principles, Wittgenstein taught his readers what language games were through various examples of language games in use. He seemingly did not want a simple definition because that would contradict his very point. We understand language from how we use it, not from definitions. Some examples of language games (which the SFBT co-founders cite later on) are:

Giving orders, and acting on them —
Describing an object by its appearance, or by its measurements —
Constructing an object from a description (a drawing) —
Reporting an event —
Speculating about the event —
Forming and testing a hypothesis —
Presenting the results of an experiment in tables and diagrams —
Making up a story; and reading one —
Acting in a play —
Singing rounds —
Guessing riddles —
Cracking a joke; telling one —
Solving a problem in applied arithmetic —
Translating from one language into another —
Requesting, thanking, cursing, greeting, praying (2009, p. 15)

Think of how a pun plays upon the different meanings of words in context. A word is not fixed, it has a malleable meaning in relation to other words and social uses. Using Wittgenstein's example, consider a curse word—I can think of one particular—that has many different meanings depending on its use. We do not need a doctorate in logic or philosophy to understand that, only to have lived in the world.

In Section 66, which I invoke you to read in its entirety in the endnotes, Wittgenstein went on to provide some background for his term *language game* by inviting the reader to explore what a game is in the first place. Wittgenstein observed there is no single characteristic that applies to all games, and thus chess is an entirely different game from ring-around-the-roses or baseball or the "quiet game" we play with children.

Consider, for example, the activities that we call "games." I mean board-games, card-games, ball-games, athletic games, and so on. What is common to them all? —Don't say: "They *must* have something in common, or they would not be called 'games'" —but *look and see* whether there is anything common to all. —For if you look at them, you won't see something that is common to *all*, but similarities, affinities, and a whole series of them at that. To repeat: don't think, but look![1]

(Section 66, p. 36)

If we try to think of one defining characteristic all games share, we will inevitably fail. Even the often-guessed feature of games as entertaining is disputed (see endnote). So there is no one unifying characteristic, yet we still know what a game is. How is this possible?

According to Wittgenstein, we were trained as to what qualifies as a game and what does not by being given countless examples of things that are labeled games and not-games throughout our lifetime. It is critical to Wittgenstein that his readers see how we are trained (in use), not explained (in dictionaries), as to what "games" are. Compare the notoriously boring video *game* "Waiting in Line 3-D" to the widely enjoyed roller-coaster, understood as a *not-game*. We could spend days trying to draw distinguishing boundaries in hindsight, but Wittgenstein argued that even if we were to do so, that is not how we came to understand game and not-game. Games crisscross and overlap each other across categories and lack precise boundaries.

Words are used in *living*, in *activities*. There is no absolute rule that governs words, only recognizable use in context. Language games refer to the particular contextual domain. Each context has its own rules that govern our use of a word in that context. Wittgenstein encouraged us to see how we use a certain word(s) in one sphere of life but use the same word(s) differently in another sphere. "Evidence" means one thing in a legal language game and another in a scientific language game. "Sick" means one thing in a medical language game and another in a skateboard language game. Language, to Wittgenstein, cannot be absolute; it must be contextualized within social activity.

Family resemblances

Wittgenstein continued his questioning: So how do we know games all belong to the same group if there is not one unifying feature? Wittgenstein's answer is that we can identify similarities between members of the group without one feature becoming the defining characteristic of all members. He termed this *family resemblances*. Some games resemble others, but a single trait does not define the group. If we were to explain what a game is to a child or adult, we would inevitably fall back upon family resemblances instead of universal explanations: "This *and similar things* are called 'games'" (p. 37). He continued:

> And do we know any more ourselves? Is it just that we can't tell others exactly what a game is? —But this is not ignorance. We don't know the boundaries because none have been drawn…. One can say that the concept of a game is a concept with blurred edges (p. 38).

TABLE 8.1 Demonstration of language games

Word	Language Game	Dominant Meaning
Sick	Medical Language Game	"Ill"
Sick	Skateboarding Language Game	"Impressive"
Cool	Slang Language Game	"Excellent"
Cool	Weather Reporting Language Game	"Moderately Cold Temperature"
Gay	1930s US Culture	"Happy"
Gay	1960s US Culture	"Homosexual" (deviant)
Gay	1970s+ US Culture (varies)	"Same-gender attraction" (self-identification and pride)

See PBS, 2024; Peters, 2014

Wittgenstein concluded that even if the concept of a game does not have clear, firm boundaries, we can still use the word and know what each other is talking about. His question of what a game is showed how we *see* the answer before we think through how we arrived at our answer.

Wittgenstein emphasized that understanding a language game is rooted in our experiences and the conventional usage of certain terms within specific communities, cultures, and areas of life. He argued that language, like games, operates based on a set of rules and we use these contextualized-language-usage situations in regular life such that it is senseless to analyze outside of our social activities, situated in different domains of life. Language—including nonverbal language—is communal communication that abides by customs and norms, and it is always a social, dynamic practice within a particular sphere. This broader cultural sphere is what Wittgenstein called a *form of life*. For example, the legal language game takes place within a form of life: a courtroom setting. The medical language game takes place within a different form of life: a hospital setting.

Wittgenstein contended that there is no way we can separate our use of language from the way we were trained to use language in a particular context. All language lies within a particular framework, and we cannot isolate it. Thus even if a word or phrase is the same, the context changes the meaning of the word or phrase. The now-dated

TABLE 8.2 Demonstration of language games and forms of life

Word	Language Game	Form of Life	Dominant Meaning
Sick	Medical Language Game	Hospital Setting	"Ill"
Sick	Skateboarding Language Game	Skate Park	"Impressive"
Cool	Slang Language Game	Social Setting	"Excellent"
Cool	Weather Reporting Language Game	News/Media	"Moderately cold temperature"
Mouse	Technology Language Game	Office Setting	"Computer device"
Mouse	Biology Language Game	Laboratory	"Rodent used for research"
Mouse	Children's Literature Language Game	Kindergarten Reading	"An anthropomorphized hero"
Mouse	Home Maintenance Language Game	Household	"Pest"
Bark	Dog Care Language Game	Dog Ownership	"The sound a dog makes"
Bark	Botany Language Game	Forest	"The outer layer of a tree"
Gay	Early 20th Century US Cultural Language Game	Social Setting	"Happy"
Gay	Modern-Day US Social Identity Language Game	Social Setting	"A Person Attracted To People Of The Same Gender"

childhood literary character Amelia Bedelia comes to mind. Amelia is instructed to "draw the drapes" and proceeds to draw a picture of curtains hanging over the windows; however, this is not what the speaker meant. The speaker intended for Amelia to close the curtains. This book series was meant to help facilitate childhood reading comprehension. It highlighted the peculiar characteristics of language. I think Wittgenstein would have liked the intention behind these books and would have pointed out that Amelia is not wrong, just not matching language games with the speaker. They are misaligned. Wittgenstein adamantly opposed the idea of a privileged or superior language game; he emphasized that different language games provide distinct settings for language, each with its own internal coherence and validity (Cockburn, 2023).

My students often resonate with the following thought experiment as an example. Two friends are out for a walk in December. One person says, "It's freezing out!" to indicate they are cold during their winter stroll. Their companion, well-versed in scientific language games, replies, "To freeze is to change from a liquid to a solid. Assuming we are talking about water, we would have to have 0 degrees Celsius and 1,013 millibars of pressure for it to be freezing." The friend is employing a scientific language game to make meaning of the words, one of chemistry to be specific. However, this was not the language game the speaker intended. Consequently, these two friends are missing each other's meaning, ending up in what Wittgenstein termed *non-sense*. I find it important to reiterate that Wittgenstein would not denounce either speaker for being wrong. The takeaway is not that one person is mistaken. The takeaway is that both are caught in a misunderstanding because of the idiosyncrasies of our language. The example above highlights how the friends are in this confusing predicament because our language is far from objective and in no way depictive of reality. Meaning can and must be found in usage—in life.

Private language

To reiterate, words and concepts shape the way we think, but this is not due to the inherent logical principles of language (as previous philosophers, logicians, and linguists contended) but rather to their usage based on a particular language game in a particular form of life. Since language loses coherence if separated from its language game and viewed in isolation, we must acknowledge the need for social agreement in how words are used within specific practices. This is the "training" Wittgenstein talks about.

Remember that Wittgenstein did not believe one language game should be privileged over another. Attempting to describe our experiences in the world solely through a scientific language game as though it were the only language game that matters leads to confusion and false propositions and conclusions. This is a significant point and is worth re-reading. This is also a necessary point to understand Wittgenstein's *private language argument*.

Wittgenstein believed a *private language* was ridiculous. Individual "inner" (i.e., private) sensations and experiences can never be *known*. According to Wittgenstein, there is no knowing but only *experiencing* private sensations such as moods or pain. When you stub your toe, you say, "Ouch!"—or some other word. Presumably, you said this immediately and did not pause to consider, "Is this pain? It might not be. Well, yes, now that I have thought about it, I know this is pain." Wittgenstein pointed out our ludicrous use of language about *knowing* pain because *to know* implies *to doubt*, and we never doubt that we are in pain. Our inner thoughts, moods, feelings, and sensations are for us alone to *experience*, not *know*. Our private experiences are just that— private; meanwhile, language and thus meaning are inherently communal. Basically, if we can talk about it, it is not private; if we cannot talk about it, it is not sensical language, and, being unintelligible to anyone, it cannot be a language. I suggest you re-read this paragraph a couple of times until it makes at least some sense. de Shazer was very taken with this idea, as you will see in the next chapter.

Wittgenstein offered an example about private experiences I imagine most of us have thought about at some point in our lives. What one person experiences as "red" may be entirely different from how another experiences red. Maybe what I see as "red" looks like what I would call "green" to you. It may be the case that each person has their own red experience, but, as Wittgenstein emphasized, nobody can ever *know* whether other people see their red or another red. It is simply impossible to cross-check our inner experiences of red (see p. 102). Wittgenstein further argued that just because we cannot verify your red = my red, the word "red" can still be used in our daily lives. This concept is also illustrated by his famous metaphor of a beetle in a box.[2] You can find this complete entry in the endnotes.

Suppose that everyone had a box with something in it which we call a "beetle." No one can ever look into anyone else's box, and everyone says he knows what a beetle is only by looking at his beetle. —Here, it would be quite possible for everyone to have something different in his box. One might even imagine such a thing constantly changing. —But what if these people's word "beetle" had a *use* nonetheless?

(p. 106, italics added for emphasis)

Instead of focusing on the "fact" of what the beetle *is*, Wittgenstein pointed out we can focus on the utility of having a word to communicate with others within a language game. Thus, Wittgenstein believed it was important for us to become more attentive to our language games and less attached to the idea that humans can know everything as an absolute picture or idea if we just think hard enough over a long enough time period. We cannot know another's red, and we cannot know another's beetle. The same goes for the private experience I might term "depression." How do I know my experience that I call "depression" matches what you call "depression?" Wittgenstein argued that you cannot *know* inner states, only experience them.

Furthermore, why, Wittgenstein probed, would we waste our time trying to get an ultimate definition of "red," "depression," or whatever the beetle in the box might be? There is no way to *know* because there is no way to *check*. And really, is that really the best use of the greatest minds? Where would such thinking really get us?

As you can read in the endnotes, *Philosophical Investigations* highlighted the glaring mistake people make by thinking in the following way: as physics is to matter and energy, so is psychology to inner states.[3] The physicist "sees, hears, thinks about, and informs us of these phenomena; and the psychologist observes the utterances (the behavior) of the subject" (p. 159). A rock falling from a cliff can be directly observed;

however, a mental state is not directly observable. He argued it is the client's *language* that is observed: how they describe "depression" through words and nonverbal language, which is secondary. Therefore, Wittgenstein entreated psychology (used as an umbrella term for all mental health practices) to pay attention to language games rather than imagining they know clients' feelings, pains, moods, states, or other private experiences.

The *Philosophical Investigations* is an experience I would argue one has to undergo themselves—at least in part—to really *see* SFBT. This book is a collection of scattered lecture notes and other thoughts that were later brought together and numbered. The sections are themed but do not progress with deductive reasoning such as the example, "Socrates is a man. All men are mortal. Therefore, Socrates is mortal." There is more of an argument to be made that Wittgenstein used inductive reasoning because worked from specific examples to larger generalizations at times. However, attempting to neatly categorize Wittgenstein overlooks his unique philosophical method.

Wittgenstein's book is not an explanation or description. The *Investigations* is a journey. It is an erratic part-conversation, and one he was not even sure he wanted published. Wittgenstein taught his readers through examples which contained artificial dialogues with an unknown other, so he presented his points as dialogical demonstrations rather than presenting his work as a whole in a conventional sense. I believe it is best that my readers read *Philosophical Investigations* for themselves. It would be inconsistent with Wittgenstein's philosophy to assume, even with all the time in the world, that I could convey his meaning rather than have an individual *experience* it.

SUMMARY

Wittgenstein was an atheoretical philosopher who abandoned his earlier position that words are pictures of reality. His later philosophy impressed upon others the importance of culture, relationships, and context. He believed we already know what language is because we use it every day, and there is no need to analyze language like a scientist trying to show atomistic constituent components. Wittgenstein was against the reification of Science (capital "S") in religion, philosophy, psychology, and other arenas in which he thought we were mismatching language games without realizing it. Having an engineering background, he appreciated science but did not appreciate the scientification of the non-scientific. Wittgenstein highlighted that in science, you can explain or say, but in other contexts, such as moods, pain, art, or music, you can only *show*. Rather than searching for an explanatory characteristic, it would be enough to accept family resemblances. There is so much we *see* but cannot *say*.

Wittgenstein's approach to philosophy was novel in that it paid unique attention to language and meaning in relation to a social world governed by cultural conventions and rules. His way of thinking was unlike previous renowned philosophers and linguists, and he made huge waves at Cambridge. He contested the dominant views of language either in isolation, as a static thing, and/or as representational of the world.

Wittgenstein's concepts—especially those of language games, family resemblances, and private language—impacted many postmodern thinkers across disciplines. His work, particularly his later work exhibited in *Philosophical Investigations*, had major influences on postmodern family therapy founders Steve de Shazer, Insoo Kim Berg, Michael White, and Harlene Anderson. One can find bits of Wittgenstein's ideas in SFBT, narrative therapy, and collaborative-dialogic practices; however, I argue that Wittgenstein had the greatest impact on Steve de Shazer and Insoo Kim Berg (the co-founders of SFBT).

REFLECTIVE QUESTIONS

1. Can you think of some examples of language games?
2. Can you think of examples of different forms of life?
3. How does meaning change based on language games and forms of life?
4. What is Wittgenstein's private language argument?
5. How does his private language argument relate to psychology and psychotherapy?

Keywords

Language Games
Family Resemblances
Forms of Life
Private Language

Ludwig Wittgenstein Post-Test (Inspired by Student Questions)

1. How did Wittgenstein challenge the idea that there is a fixed meaning for words?
   a. Wittgenstein highlighted that we know what a word means from living in a society where we are trained as to when to use certain words and in what contexts. He did not think we know what a word means by looking it up in the dictionary because there is no fixed meaning that is constant across all contexts.
2. Did Wittgenstein believe in an objective reality?
   a. This answer is tricky, and commentators will respond with conflicting answers. Wittgenstein's *Philosophical Investigations* actually included the famous image of the duck-rabbit. If you looked at it one way, you saw a clear drawing of a duck, however, if you looked at it slightly differently, you saw a clear drawing of a rabbit. If he did believe in an objective reality, he believed that language and interpretation were strong enough factors to offer multiple contradictory perspectives at once. Most scholars agree that Wittgenstein's philosophy is skeptical of applying positivist principles to language. Everything depends on how you look at it (and how you language it).
3. What did Wittgenstein believe was the relationship of language to reality?
   a. Early-Wittgenstein believed in the "picture theory" that language represents reality; however, late-Wittgenstein rejected this idea. Whereas early-Wittgenstein believed words reflected the "objective" nature of reality, late-Wittgenstein questioned objectivity and believed we cannot extract language from context.

4. What was so radical about late-Wittgenstein's philosophy?

   a. Whereas most philosophers and academics saw philosophy through the lens of inductive or deductive reasoning to derive truths about our language and our world, Wittgenstein looked to the everyday use of language. He argued we already *see* meaning in our daily lives, even if it is impossible to articulate in language. So there is no such thing as the "right word" as long as people can understand what we mean. How many times have you struggled to remember the "correct" word, but your friend understood what you meant anyway? Wittgenstein's philosophy was "down to earth" in this way, focused on daily practices of living rather than Platonic ideals or logical proofs.

5. How does Wittgenstein's understanding of language compare and contrast to the cybernetic concepts of "report and command" in language?

   a. In cybernetics, "report" refers to the data or information, and "command" refers to the communication about how to interpret the report. Cybernetics focuses on report (i.e., information) and command (i.e., how to understand the information) being constitutive of communication in systems. Contrastingly, Wittgenstein thought language was like a game, so words have different meanings depending on the language game (like how "sick" has different meanings in a skateboard language game versus a medical language game). Wittgenstein's focus on language games and forms of life emphasizes language as a communal activity within a particular game set in a particular social context. Where cybernetics will focus on feedback loops on shaping interpretation and meaning, Wittgenstein would focus on socio-cultural factors and forms of life in shaping interpretation and meaning.

6. What is the meaning of Wittgenstein's quote that opens this chapter: "The question, 'What is a word really?' is analogous to, 'What is a piece in chess?'"

   a. This is often interpreted to mean that you cannot answer what a piece is because chess pieces are different (e.g., bishop versus queen), and you need to understand the entire game of chess to describe them as part of it. Different pieces serve different roles, and these roles determine a piece's meaning and function. As Wittgenstein said, "Its meaning lies in its use" (2009, p. 86).

NOTES

1 Section 66 ... —Look, for example, at board-games, with their various affinities. Now pass to card-games; here you find many correspondences with the first group, but many common features drop out, and others appear. When we pass next to ball-games, much that is common is retained, but much is lost. —Are they all *"entertaining"*? Compare chess with noughts and crosses. Or is there always winning and losing, or competition between players? Think of patience. In ball-games, there is winning and losing; but when a child throws his ball at the wall and catches it again, this feature has disappeared. Look at the parts played by skill and luck, and at the difference between skill in chess and skill in tennis. Think now of singing and dancing games; here we have the element of entertainment, but how many other characteristic features have disappeared! And we can go through the many, many other groups of games in the same way, can see how similarities crop up and disappear. And the upshot of these considerations is: we see a complicated network of similarities overlapping and criss-crossing: similarities in the large and in the small (Wittgenstein, 1953/2009, p. 36).

2 Section 293. If I say of myself that it is only from my own case that I know what the word "pain" means—must I not say that of other people too? And how can I generalize the one case so irresponsibly? Well, everyone tells me that he knows what pain is only from his own case! —Suppose that everyone had a box with something in it which we call a "beetle." No one can ever look into anyone else's box, and everyone says he knows what a beetle is only by looking at his beetle. —Here it would be quite possible for everyone to have something different in his box. One might even imagine such a thing constantly changing. —But what if these people's word "beetle" had a use nonetheless? —If so, it would not be as the name of a thing. The thing in the box doesn't belong to the language game at all; not even as a Something: for the box might even be empty. —No, one can "divide through" by the thing in the box; it cancels out, whatever it is. That is to say, if we construe the grammar of the expression of sensation on the model of "object and name," the object drops out of consideration as irrelevant (Wittgenstein, 1953/2009, pp. 106–107).

3 Section 571. A misleading parallel: psychology treats of processes in the mental sphere, as does physics in the physical. Seeing, hearing, thinking, feeling, willing are not the subject matter of psychology in the same sense as that in which the movements of bodies, the phenomena of electricity, and so forth are the subject matter of physics. You can see this from the fact that the physicist sees, hears, thinks about, and informs us of these phenomena, and the psychologist observes the utterances (the behavior) of the subject (Wittgenstein, 1953/2009, p. 159).

LUDWIG WITTGENSTEIN: PRIMARY SOURCES

Wittgenstein, L. (1922). *Tractatus logico-philosophicus*. Edinburgh Press.
Wittgenstein, L. (2009). *Philosophical investigations* (G. E. M. Anscombe, P. M. S. Hacker, & J. Schulte Trans., Rev. 4th dig. ed.). Wiley Blackwell. (Original work published 1953).

Renowned Sources

Cockburn, D. (2022). *Wittgenstein, human beings, and conversation*. Anthem Press.
Cockburn, D. (2023). Lagerspetz, Wittgenstein, and Anscombe on idealism. In J. Ahlskog, & H. Strandberg (Eds.), *Philosophy as a form of life* (pp. 10–23). Åbo Akademi University Press.
Diamond, C. (2017, April 28). *Wittgenstein changes his mind* [Lecture recording]. St. John's College. https://digitalarchives.sjc.edu/items/show/2134
Grayling, A. C. (2001). *Wittgenstein: A very short introduction*. Oxford University Press.
Hertzberg, L. (2022). *Wittgenstein and the life we live with language*. Anthem Press.
Hollingworth, M. (2018). *Ludwig Wittgenstein*. Oxford University Press.
Klagge, J. C. (2016). *Simply Wittgenstein*. Simply Charly.
Monk, R. (2019). *How to read Wittgenstein* (dig. ed.). Granta Books.
Smith, M. (2021). *Wittgenstein and the problem of metaphysics*. Bloomsbury.

Additional References

Eilenberger, W. (2020). *Time of the magicians: Wittgenstein, Benjamin, Cassirer, Heidegger, and the decade that reinvented philosophy* (S. Whiteside, Trans.). Penguin.
PBS. (2024). *History of the word 'gay" | Origin of everything* [Video]. https://gpb. pbslearningmedia.org/resource/history-of-the-word-gay-video/origin-of-everything/
Peters, J. W. (2014, March 21). The decline and fall of the "H" word. *The New York Times*. https://www.nytimes.com/2014/03/23/fashion/gays-lesbians-the-term-homosexual.html
Peters, M. A. (2019). Wittgenstein and the ethics of suicide. Homosexuality and Jewish self-hatred in find de siècle Vienna. *Educational Philosophy and Theory, 51*(10), 981–990.
Peters, M. A. (2022). Wittgenstein, mysticism and the 'religious point of view': 'Whereof one cannot speak, thereof one must be silent'. *Educational Philosophy and Theory, 54*(12), 1952–1959.

CHAPTER 9

What ideas from Wittgenstein resonated with Steve de Shazer and Insoo Kim Berg?

The path to solution talk

....

Remember, as you read through these chapters, you can always return to the Introduction to refresh your memory on the terms you learned such as epistemology, postmodernism, positivism, and post-structuralism.

QUESTIONS TO THINK ABOUT

1. What is the significance of theory in solution focused brief therapy (SFBT)?
2. What is solution talk?
3. What is a solution focused language game and why is it necessary for understanding solution talk?
4. Why was it important for the founders to address the private language argument?
5. How did Wittgenstein influence how emotions are addressed in SFBT?

Steve de Shazer and Insoo Kim Berg resonated with Ludwig Wittgenstein's concepts, particularly his later philosophy detailed in the *Philosophical Investigations*. Their adoption of his philosophy, particularly the rejection of a *private language* and the idea that meaning is co-constructed in conversation within *language games*, forms the bedrock of SFBT. These founders paid attention to grammar, language structure, and context to orient the client toward solutions instead of problems, and they focused on what was right in front of them. These founders meticulously attended to solution talk, as explained in this chapter. They emphasized the importance of what was immediately present, encapsulated in the idea that "solution focused therapy is about constructing solutions, not solving problems" (Miller & de Shazer, p. 15).

DOI: 10.4324/9781003439349-13

Perhaps related to his decision to move to Vienna in his late life, de Shazer was deeply fascinated by the Viennese philosopher and became known in the family therapy community as a Wittgensteinian scholar (de Shazer et al., 2021). de Shazer directly credited Wittgenstein as part of developing his approach in SFBT (e.g., de Shazer, 1991, p. xv; Miller & de Shazer, 2000, p. 7, 15). In his article co-authored with one of his colleagues at the BFTC, Gale Miller and he discussed late-Wittgenstein's concepts of language games and private language (Miller & de Shazer, p. 5) where he and Miller described how they believed a therapist could best implement a solution focused approach by incorporating these concepts. They used Wittgenstein's philosophy as a template for conceptualizing emotions in therapy (p. 9).

Her husband's enthusiasm for Wittgenstein influenced Berg's solution focused practice. We can find evidence of this, for instance, when she included quotes from Wittgenstein in her book about solution focused coaching (see Berg & Szabó, 2005). de Shazer and Berg adopted Wittgenstein's ideas about philosophy being an *activity* in which we are liable to become "bewitched by our language" (de Shazer et al., p. 114), and they applied this understanding to therapy (de Shazer, 1997):

> Throughout these years I have used Ludwig Wittgenstein's work as one of my tools for attempting to dismantle muddles. Recently it dawned on me that Wittgenstein repeatedly dealt with issues and concerns of philosophers that are at least as robust and overdetermined as the issues and concerns of therapists. Furthermore, it struck me that the structure of philosophical muddles is the same as the structure of therapeutic muddles. That is, both are deeply embedded in language, in the way we talk and write about things (p. 133).

THE SIGNIFICANCE OF THEORY AND PHILOSOPHY IN SFBT

Recall from Chapter 7 how Berg and de Shazer were proud of their model being created inductively, starting from practice instead of theory (Berg & Szabó, 2005). Recall in Chapter 8 that Wittgenstein's philosophy was anti-philosophical—in the traditional sense. Wittgenstein was much more interested in our everyday, practical use of language. One can see Wittgenstein's beliefs echoed in de Shazer's comment below.

> In recent years, epistemological issues have resurfaced in the field of family therapy. Too frequently the discussion of these issues has remained on a philosophical level, and therefore the practical implications of any epistemology are clothed in fog and muddle. However, consistent conceptual schemes are necessary for the development of thinking about therapy and thus the development of therapeutic methodologies.
>
> *(de Shazer, 2017, p. 72)*

This may bring up questions about just how important theory and philosophy are in this model. Luckily for us, it is unnecessary to enter a fiery debate about to what extent theory and philosophy influenced SFBT. de Shazer addressed this directly. He cleared up any seeming contradiction by explaining that SFBT does not rely on any grand theory or metanarrative (de Shazer et al.), which is a logical postmodern stance;

meanwhile, SFBT brings in Wittgenstein's "non-systematic, rambling, digressive, and subversive ways to make the reader *look again* and thus think in new and different ways" (p. 138).

Until you read Berg and de Shazer's work yourself, allow me to humbly explain the importance of "theory" in SFBT. By my count, in just one book chapter de Shazer mentioned the word *theory* or a close derivation such as *theories* or *theorist* 36 times, and he mentioned the word *philosopher* or a close derivation such as *philosophers* or *philosophies* 31 times (see de Shazer et al., Chapter 6: "Don't Think But Observe"). For a founder who was disinterested in theory or philosophy, he sure talked about it a lot. It is also interesting that the chapter's title is a play off Wittgenstein's "Don't think, but *look ... look* and *see!*" (Wittgenstein, 2009, p. 36). This is in the section of the *Philosophical Investigations* where Wittgenstein introduced language games, Section 66.

Renowned SFBT colleagues Harry Korman (who co-authored with Berg and de Shazer), Peter De Jong (who co-authored with Berg), and Sara Smock Jordan did their own digging into de Shazer's primary sources.

> de Shazer wrote 6 books and about 75 papers and at least one-third of that content is about theory. Eve Lipchik, an important early contributor to the development of SFBT, wrote about the evolution of SFBT in its first ten years: "The team [at the Brief Family Therapy Center in Milwaukee (BFTC)] always tried to use theory to guide practice and to further test theory-driven practices with clients" (Lipchik et al., 2013, p. 6). Given this close relationship of theory and practice at BFTC, the authors believe it is essential to closely examine de Shazer's "theory" in his writings to more fully understand the development of SFBT.
>
> *(Korman et al., 2020, p. 47)*

My interpretation of de Shazer's writings matches that of Korman and colleagues, namely, whether SFBT has a "theory" and how important "theory" is depends on how you define "theory" to begin with. The same goes for the word "philosophy." If you understand late-Wittgenstein's writings, the tension dissolves and de Shazer's peculiar comments begin to make sense. An example of a perplexing comment and its explanation can be found below.

Conference Attendee (to de Shazer): *"What do you do with depression?"*
de Shazer: *"I don't understand the question."* (Korman et al., p. 47)

The question, "What do you do with depression?" presupposes that a therapist *does something* with depression, which does not fit an SFBT framework. de Shazer's response, "I don't understand the question" would often lead to participants asking about his theory on depression, mental illness, or whatever. de Shazer would then respond that SFBT has no theory about those things. This and similar responses may have contributed to the belief that SFBT has no theory.

(Korman et al., p. 47)

This quote provides the context we needed to see how it makes sense that many people interested in SFBT would believe that it does not have a theory: because de Shazer said so; however, since they did not understand Wittgenstein, they did not understand de Shazer's language game. Wittgenstein/de Shazer had no theory about depression and so on because that would require a grand, theoretical explanation.

Think of it this way: Wittgenstein's philosophy is anti-philosophy, and his theory is anti-theory. We must avoid conflating "Theory" with "theory." As Korman et al. explained, SFBT disregards a grand Theory *as part of its theory*. Similarly, Berg and her colleague Szabó described it as "a theory of no Theory" (p. 15).

> Theory, research/search, and practice all guide, influence, and change each other. For example, a change in practice (if it is a difference that seems to make a difference) will suggest a new area for disciplined observation (or search), which, in turn, will send the theorist to the library looking for a frame or frames to help them describe things in a clear and useful manner. What is developed is certainly not a Theory with a capital T; rather, the analysis leads away from such a grand design, emphasizing instead the variability of the clinical situation and the people involved, the variability of events, and the variability of problems and solutions.
>
> *(de Shazer, 1991, p. xx)*

If we can agree that Theory (capital "T") and Philosophy (capital "P") are no longer useful according to a solution focused conceptualization, we are left with the theory(/philosophy) of valuing practicality and usefulness over Theory. This crosses over with a broader, post-structuralist understanding (see de Shazer & Berg, 1992).

LANGUAGE AS AN ACTIVITY

Many scholars describe Wittgenstein's work along the lines of: "not a body of doctrine but an *activity*" (e.g., Monk, 2019, p. vii). de Shazer and Berg continuously described therapeutic work as an *activity*, in a Wittgensteinian sense of attending to language (e.g., Berg & de Shazer, 1993). As de Shazer (2005) explained, "Language is an activity within specific contexts, not something captured in dictionaries and grammar books. Words are defined by how two or more people, in a particular context, use them" (p. 1). Wittgenstein's influence explains why SFBT is not a fixed set of techniques or doctrines but an ongoing, dynamic, conversational process.

Language games

de Shazer offered multiple descriptions of *language games* such as "slices of everyday life" (de Shazer et al., p. 110) and "the various, organized ways in which we use language to get things done" (Miller & de Shazer, 2000, p. 8). He used an example of "stealing" in baseball versus "stealing" a car (de Shazer, 2005, p. 1). But perhaps my favorite description of language games is in de Shazer and Berg's (1992) article:

> A language game is an *activity* seen as a language complete in itself, a complete system of human communication. You've got what you've got, and that's all

there is. There is no need to look behind or beneath since everything you need is readily available and open to view. *Nothing is hidden.*

(p. 75, italics added for emphasis)

Their co-authored article centered around "the fact that *doing* therapy involves using language" (p. 71), and they challenged traditional therapeutic understandings, shifting the focus from a search for a problematic root cause to "*doing* therapy" (p. 71). They pointed out that family therapists and other mental health practitioners have historically attended less to the interactional way in which we use language than to a positivist, "scientific" view. According to de Shazer and Berg (1992), that language is accurate, reliable, or stable is merely a comforting daydream:

We all would like language to behave itself, to be precise. This is particularly so in a field such as psychotherapy or family therapy which we think of as somehow being "scientific" or at least involving more than everyday rigor in the use of language. When we use and hear the words "rigor" or "scientific language," we credit such language with greater reliability. These beliefs are useful because they help us maintain (at least) the illusion that there is a semblance of order, logic, and/or (at least) consistency in our world. However, our experience suggests that language is not so precise, logical, or consistent (pp. 71–72).

Building on their critique of positivism, Berg and de Shazer argued that language should be understood within the context of meaning and use. Just as Wittgenstein said there was no ultimate language game that topped all others, the SFBT founders agreed there was no reason scientific knowledge should take precedence over all other language games (1992, p. 74). They provided an example from the television show *All in the Family.*

Edith Bunker asks Archie if he would like his new bowling shoes laced right over left or left over right. Archie asks, "What's the difference?" Edith then begins to explain how lacing the shoes right over left is different from lacing the shoes left over right. As she explains, Archie gets more and more frustrated and angry and tries to get Edith to explain to him just exactly "What's the difference?" (p. 72)

Recalling my earlier thought experiment about the conversation between two friends about whether it was freezing outside, we can apply the founders' example in the same way. This is Berg and de Shazer's illustration of the same misunderstanding: the confusion that comes from mixing up our language games. As Wittgenstein himself would have pointed out, and I hope I have shown with my example, de Shazer and Berg emphasized that neither party is right nor wrong here. Both interpretations are valid according to our language: "In different language games, the 'same' word may have different uses and therefore different meanings" (p. 76). Since either interpretation is valid, we immediately see there is no absolute meaning that words carry with them. Recognizing this, Miller and de Shazer discussed how different therapy models themselves will use different language games, "each involving a somewhat different vocabulary and grammar for talking about clients' lives and troubles and how change happens" (2000, p. 8).

Applying this to an SFBT session, we need not spend time chasing down what the client *really* means, because we can *see* what they are from the context. Remember, *nothing is hidden*. Essentially, stop hunting for Truth in therapeutic conversations. "Meanings are open to view since they lie in between people rather than hidden away inside an individual (psyche, system, family structure, etc.)" (p. 74).

A SHORT REFLECTION ON LANGUAGE GAMES IN SFBT

In his discussion on scaling questions, de Shazer said, "Remember, 'Feeling better' is not necessarily the same as 'Feeling good.' 'Feeling good' is from a different language game" (2005, p. 7). This indeed is a helpful reminder that we receive answers to the questions we ask. After reading this chapter, you will see how the parameters of a conversation shape the outcome of that conversation.

A SOLUTION-FOCUSED LANGUAGE GAME

We have now reached the heart and soul of SFBT: what de Shazer and Berg called a *solution-focused language game* (1992, p. 77). To me, having an understanding of what de Shazer and Berg meant by a solution-focused language game demonstrates an understanding of how to integrate theory and practice in SFBT. Since language is a communal activity and cannot take place in isolation, a solution-focused language game would structure the grammar of the conversation in such a way that it created specific, contextual "rules" for how language was to be used.

Berg and de Shazer used solution-focused language games to recontextualize and reword the clients' language around a particular problem. Their solution-focused language game created an idea of impermanence and underscored a conceptualization of each presenting problem as solvable. From this perspective, the problem becomes workable through language, and change is possible. The key is to use what is right in front of you. Again, *nothing is hidden*. See if you can make sense of de Shazer's (1997) grammatical illustration below:

Compare—
I am male. | He is a male.
I am an American. | He is an American.
I am a schizophrenic. | He is a schizophrenic.
What happens in the third sentence? Remember the DSM (Diagnostic and Statistical Manual of Mental Disorders) and the long tradition of diagnosis in psychiatry. The "is" in all three sentences using the third-person singular involves the same grammatical form of identity (2×2 is 4).
Compare—
2×2 is 4. | He = schizophrenic.
The rose is red. | Rose = + red.
The grammar of the "is" in the second sentence (about a rose) is different. Here the verb is something that bonds two different things together. Our grammar leads us, naturally, to the conclusion that schizophrenia is incurable: once a schizophrenic, always a schizophrenic. We do not need psychiatry or even Theory for this, just grammar.

...

I am an alcoholic. | He is an alcoholic.

What happens here? Evidently, AA (Alcoholics Anonymous), like psychiatry (with schizophrenia), is seduced by the verb "to be" into believing that an alcoholic is a steady state; something permanent. This leads to the idea that in spite of 30 years without a drink, he is still a (recovering!) alcoholic! The "is" within this mythology is in fact so strong that probably no empirical evidence will influence AA or the diagnostic language game. (p. 135)

...

Compare—

I feel better. | I am better.

You feel better. | You are better.

He feels better. | He is better. (p. 141)

At the start of sessions, a solution focused therapist shifts away from "I am" such as the example, "I am an alcoholic." Later, the therapist will come back to "I am" to solidify the changes the client has made, "taking advantage of the grammar" (p. 141), such as can be found in the example: "I am better." A solution focused brief therapist might exclaim, "Wow! It is clear that *you are* better!" (p. 41).

Language games cannot be separated from personal, everyday living nor professional, psychotherapeutic work (e.g., a solution-focused language game or a diagnostic language game). The example above illustrates the consequences of the structure of our language. How many solutions can we construct just by changing our grammar? An adept solution focused therapist finds opportunities to use language as a resource and to create useful shifts in clients' language (de Shazer, 1997). "The solution focused therapy language game is a distinctive strategy for constructing change in therapy which requires that solution focused therapists adopt a different orientation than other therapists" (Miller & de Shazer, p. 15). And it is not just solutions that are being constructed, but also realities (Hoyt, 1996).

A scaling language game

As de Shazer (2005) described, he came up with scaling questions organically in a conversation with a client who said they felt "better but not a perfect 10" (p. 2).

In this particular scaling language game, "10" is defined, perhaps, as "perfect" although we never talked about this definition. Regardless of how we might have defined "10," he felt better than how he had felt in years, and "8.5" is defined as "not a perfect 10." The client and I now have established a language game in which both "better" and "worse" are easily referred to simply with a single digit (p. 2).

Let us go through Wittgenstein/de Shazer's views line by line. (1) There is no such thing as an absolute definition because words are not representational of reality, so there doesn't have to be a so-called proper definition of "10." To try to find an absolute definition would be preposterous and a waste of time; it is not necessary for their purpose. (2) It is only important that they understand one another, so how they use language in their shared context is what is important. From the context they created, it is obvious that 8.5 does not equal 10, and that numbers nearer to 10 are preferable. That is as much as we need to know. Remember, *"Nothing is hidden"* (de Shazer & Berg, 1992, p. 75). (3) Language games are contexts in which we understand the language that we use. de Shazer said, "By using the term 'game' Wittgenstein emphasizes the fact that language is like a game and that, like many games, there are rules involved and often multiple players" (p. 2). It is like an inside joke. The participants are using language in a particular way, governed by the unspoken rules they created. They each *see* what the other means. And now they have a short-hand way of speaking. In summary, a scaling language game is not meant to be an objective measurement. But it has a use nonetheless.

A miracle question language game

Another useful language game developed over 20 years ago when my colleagues and I picked up the idea of using the concept of miracles from our clients. One day a client was asked: "How will you know that this problem is gone?" She responded, "That would take a miracle!" The therapist, Insoo Kim Berg, then said, "Well, suppose that a miracle did happen. What would be different?" From there the client and therapist were able to develop a picture of how the client's life would be different if a miracle were to happen.

(de Shazer, 2005, p. 2)

de Shazer explained that the SFBT miracle language game situates "miracle" in a different language game and is not meant to be used in a religious language game. The miracle question language game provides a framework for exploring new, possible futures. It provides the parameters of the conversation and shifts the focus away from the problem and toward solutions.

Like the scaling question language game, the point is that the client and therapist develop their own rules of the conversation in which they understand one another and co-develop meaning. By employing the miracle language game, the client and therapist develop a unique understanding of what progress would be. There is no objective measurement that makes the miracle concrete. The miracle is fleshed out through the conversation whereby the client provides details and descriptions, but these are neither interpreted as universal nor generalized. Every miracle is different.

Solution talk

"Solution talk" is the main solution-focused language game. More than a mere technique, this language game sets the parameters of how to have an SFBT conversation. Solution talk is a language game that (re)frames all solution-focused questions, allowing therapists to shift how a problem is seen and talked about (de Shazer, 1991).

In contrast to solution talk, there is *"problem talk,"* another language game that keeps the focus on the problem and failed solution attempts or what has not been working. Problem talk perpetuates what led the client to seek therapy, as it does not contribute to constructing solutions (Berg & de Shazer, 1993). To be concise about the difference between these two language games, "Problem talk creates problems, solution talk creates solutions" (de Shazer as cited in Berg & Szabó, 2005, p. 11). SFBT is rooted in the construction of solutions rather than the resolution of problems (Miller & de Shazer, p. 15).

Solution talk introduces hope and change by implying that problems are fleeting and that solutions are within reach. By using solution talk, the therapist and client work together to find solutions that work for them. These solutions can be identified by looking at exceptions to the problem or using the imagination of a miracle to gather momentum on actionable steps clients can take.

Berg and de Shazer noted that clients often entered the therapy room assuming a problem-focused language game (i.e., problem talk). SFBT therapists would want to pay extra attention to active listening and introducing subtle language shifts to transition to solution talk (de Shazer & Berg, 1992; de Shazer et al., 2021).

> The language used for solution development differs significantly from that needed to describe a problem. Problem talk tends to be negative and past-focused and often suggests the permanence of a problem. In contrast, the language of solutions is usually more positive, hopeful, and future-focused, and suggests the transience of problems.
>
> *(de Shazer et al., 2021, p. 3)*

Staying grounded in solution talk, the therapist implies that the problem will no longer be a problem in the future (Miller & de Shazer). SFBT therapists avoid spending too much time on the problem, as this would change the language game. By employing solution talk, the therapist can reframe problems, using grammar to create linguistic structure alterations and change meanings (de Shazer et al., 2021, p. 3). The SFBT therapist shifts from language that focuses on the past and what went wrong to language that focuses on the present, future, and what can go right.

Some books may offer you examples of questions, but these questions are asking something different and are used as aids to help beginning therapists practice solution talk. However, if you are trying to "do" SFBT, you will need to think about Wittgenstein's influence of language games instead of a CBT-like emphasis on a recipe. In other words, stop thinking that SFBT therapists ask specific questions, and start realizing that SFBT therapists ask questions in specific ways. Once this makes sense, you are surely on the right track to "doing" SFBT.

de Shazer et al. gave us the following examples:

- "So, what is better, even a little bit, since the last time we met?" (p. 12)
- "What is the first thing Andrew will notice about you that first morning after the miracle that tells him you are feeling better without you telling him about it?" (p. 48)
- "So, what have you done that prevented things from getting worse?" (p. 61)
- "When was the last time parts of the miracle happened—even a little, tiny bit?" (p. 62)
- "6-7—so a couple of steps better than last time. So—what else is better?" (p. 70)

Solution talk keeps the conversation focused on resolution by careful attention to questions. Berg and Szabó (2005) talked about "empowering the client to be the first person to find solutions, rather than dwelling on and suffering from the problem" (p. 111) and mentioned the following examples as applied to a case of a disgruntled chef who felt underappreciated:

- Suppose I ask your boss what he appreciates the most about your work as the executive dining room chef. Any ideas about what he would say?
- I am sure you are very creative with your cooking. So what would your boss say he would like to see you become better at?
- When you "learn to control your emotions better," who would be the first to notice that you are doing it?
- So what would they see in you instead? (p. 112)

SFBT therapists utilize solution talk to effect change and help clients envision a future free from their current problems. As a student pointed out, likely not even realizing how right they were, learning SFBT is like learning a new language: "What has already been working or improved since last week" rather than, "What's been going on since last week?" (where clients are more likely to use problem talk) (see Reiter, 2023).

Solution talk begets strengths and resources. Even the well-known pre-session change assumes a solution talk stance: "What has been better since you made your appointment with us?" By punctuating conversations with enthusiasm and support for signs of solutions through means such as complimenting (de Shazer, 1982), asking coping questions for how clients have managed so far (Berg, 1994), finding exceptions to the problem (Berg, 1994), scaling progress (Berg & de Shazer, 1993), and using the miracle question to work with achievable goals (de Shazer, 1988), SFBT therapists can keep solution talk at the forefront.

PHILOSOPHY AND PSYCHOLOGY

de Shazer and collaborators (2021) talked about philosophy and its "offshoot," psychology (p. 139). As Wittgenstein had pointed out before him, de Shazer commented on how most philosophers and psychologists (in this case referring to mental health practitioners in general) mistakenly focused on trying to identify a unified characteristic of a thing. They criticized Socrates for his search for a word's essence as well as for Freud's process: a search for a root cause. de Shazer quoted Wittgenstein: "The classifications made by philosophers and psychologists are like those that someone would give who tried to classify clouds by their shape" (p. 140). de Shazer shared Wittgenstein's discontentment with Freud and Socrates for their similar use of generalization which resulted in them missing what was present in front of them for the sake of a mission to find absolute essences and causes.

de Shazer had the same three-fold complaint about Freud as Wittgenstein: (1) Freud used generalization from a specific case to all cases in psychotherapeutic practice, and (2) Freud was not open to correction, steadfastly holding the audacious position that what he was doing was "scientific" (p. 144), and (3) Freud purported that mental health professionals need an absolute explanation to be able to help others. Are all dreams wish fulfillments? Are all cases of "hysteria" the same? Can psychotherapists not practice until *the* root explanation is identified? The framework of Freud's theory ends up becoming limiting rather than insightful. As de Shazer contended: "Something is wrong here. As Sherlock Holmes would say, facts can (do, should) change theory but theory does not—should not, must not—change facts" (p. 144).

Unsurprisingly, de Shazer disdained any attempts at causality-defined practices which, he believed, took everything out of context.

> Philosophers, psychologists, and therapists constantly see the method of science as a model and are thus tempted ("tempted" is not really a strong enough word!) to ask questions and seek answers in the way science does. Perhaps because of the scientific model, we almost feel compelled to study language as an abstract system rather than as an activity. This preoccupation with and devotion to the method of science leads philosophers and therapists to desire and even demand that "the explanation of natural phenomena [be reduced] to the smallest number of primitive natural laws" (Wittgenstein, 1958, p. 18) via unified concepts and simple causal connections.
>
> *(de Shazer et al., 2021, p. 149)*

Instead of causality, de Shazer focused on context. As de Shazer informed his readers, "Understanding a sentence is much more akin to understanding a theme in music" (Wittgenstein, 1958, Section 527, as cited in de Shazer et al., 2021, p. 148). A musical note within a symphony, de Shazer maintained, must be situated in some way in relation to the other notes, and the surrounding context, to have meaning. "Similarly," he said, "when words and sentences are removed from their home—a language game or the everyday activity of speaking a language—their meaning can easily get lost" (p. 149). Social, everyday practices become a therapist's focus, and the therapist attunes to the language the client uses. Thanks especially to de Shazer, the practice of SFBT attends to a Wittgensteinian emphasis on grammar and "untying knots" (p. 148) through language.

The private language argument

As you have learned from the earlier discussion on *Philosophical Investigations*, Wittgenstein (2009) explained that a *private language* refers to sensations (p. 95), feelings (p. 95), states of consciousness (p. 3), and moods (p. 95)—an individual's private, internal experiences—embedded in a language they alone can understand. However, he quickly challenged the idea of a private language based on his view of language as a social activity. He thought it would be absurd to "accurately" describe something internal (e.g., feelings) via an external, social description (i.e., language) and consider this sensical. It was paradoxical, and you could never know if you were "right" in such a ridiculous context.

Remember that others cannot access the "S" sensation directly, outside of a social language. Even to say "has" + "sensation" to describe an inner process that is yet unnamed is still in language (Wittgenstein, 2009, p. 99). As de Shazer put it, "How were we taught this word 'depression?' I certainly did not learn it as a child by being shown a 'depression'" (de Shazer, 1997, p. 136). To be clear, the private language argument does not mean we do not experience pain, only that we need language to be able to talk about "pain" meaningfully. Although we may use language that implies otherwise, it is nonsensical to claim to know someone else's pain. Their private sensations and emotions are only known to us one step removed.

> Even when working with problems involving such apparently internal, private experiences as emotional states, SFBT therapists typically use outward criteria (scales and observable behaviors designated by the client). Following Wittgenstein's practice of focusing on external rather than internal criteria to signify change is a radical departure, not just from Freud, but from Western philosophical traditions.
>
> *(de Shazer et al., p. 181)*

The founders' understanding of the private language argument can help psychotherapists who work with clients' inner states (e.g., emotions) by being cognizant of their therapeutic language game as shaping those emotions rather than a pursuit of objectivity. Instead of meaning lying in a perceived isolation *within* us, it lies *externally* in language, contextualized in a specific language game. In other words, "the meaning of a word is in its use" (Wittgenstein, 1968, as cited in de Shazer and Berg, p. 73). The SFBT founders de Shazer and Berg tried to simplify this idea for readers when they said, "Wittgenstein's private language argument only says that we cannot speak about private experiences, our personal constructions of reality, without a public framework, without a language game" (1992, p. 76).

In Miller and de Shazer's article, de Shazer discussed a shift in Wittgenstein's writing that resonated with him, namely "Wittgenstein's practice of focusing on external rather than internal criteria to signify change" which "is a radical departure, not just from Freud, but from Western philosophical traditions" (2000, p. 181). You can compare Miller and de Shazer's version to the full excerpt of de Shazer and colleagues' (2021) version of the endnotes.[1]

> Suppose that Steve experienced a private—inner—sensation, one that he had never experienced before and for which he had no name. So Steve wrote down the letter "S" on a piece of paper to remind himself of the sensation. When the sensation happened again [and again], he wrote another "S" on the piece of paper ... until he had filled a small notebook. Now suppose Steve decides to show you, explaining he wants to share his "S" experience with you. You carefully look at the string of "S's" that goes on for page after page. You want to make sense of them in order to imagine what "S" must feel like and to share Steve's experience with him. But this is a private and fully internal sensation, one that only Steve has had and which is not marked by any external signs other than "S." How can you make sense of it? All you know is that Steve calls it "S." How can you imagine what "S" feels like since it is internal? Like you, Steve has no external or independent sources for verifying his impressions and memory of the sensations. Given these difficulties, it would be reasonable for you and Steve to declare that, despite your best efforts, you cannot share Steve's "S" experience with him and that he can never be fully certain that all of his sensations were "really" "S's" [rather than "R's" or "T's"].
>
> *(Miller & de Shazer, p. 10)*

Compare this to Wittgenstein's musings:

> How do words *refer* to sensations? —How is the connection between the name and the thing named set up? This question is the same as: How does a human being learn the meaning of names of sensations? For example, of the word 'pain.' How can I even attempt to interpose language between the expression of pain and the pain?
>
> *(Wittgenstein, 2009, p. 95)*

Borrowing Wittgenstein's example,[2] de Shazer highlighted how the "S" thought experiment demonstrated how we do not have access to *knowledge about* our private feelings, states, and moods. We have our own *experiences* of private feelings, states, and moods. As Wittgenstein pointed out in his argument against a private language, we can never share inner processes except through outward criteria. Miller and de Shazer elaborated upon using examples such as blushing or tears as a start (p. 183).

Further expounding upon Wittgenstein's private language argument, de Shazer challenged the view that we can know someone is happy in the way they experience a state of happiness. Instead of knowing someone is happy, de Shazer argued that we can see external criteria that indicate to us that someone is happy such as a smile or laugh. We call that knowing someone is happy, but we do not have direct access to their inner experiences. "Wittgenstein suggests that an important question about feelings, such as feeling better, is: 'In what sort of context does it occur?'" (de Shazer et al., p. 113).

The same can be said for other feelings such as feeling angry or anxious: "He is scowling and therefore we say, 'He feels angry,' and he is rapidly pacing back and forth and therefore we say, 'He feels anxious'" (p. 184). We need to ask the person, "Do you feel X?" to verify whether we are right. Contrast this to your own experience of these feelings; de Shazer said that for one to say, "I feel angry" or "I feel anxious" is much closer to saying "Ouch!" than a form of knowledge that one could doubt (p. 185). This is de Shazer's summary of Wittgenstein's private language argument: there is no way for someone to "have special private knowledge about their own inner states and processes. In order for us to talk about, make sense of, and perhaps define, these inner processes, we need outward criteria that can be referenced and shared with others" (p. 183). In a therapeutic context, the private language argument means it is impossible for either the client or therapist to "really know" what's going on inside a client. The outward criteria give us a starting point, however, to ask questions. If we see a smile, we might ask, "Are you happy?" If we see tears, we might ask, "Are you sad?" And if we see a grimace, we might ask, "Are you angry?" As cited in de Shazer and Berg (1992, p. 71), "Our mistake is to look for an explanation where we ought to look at what happens" (Wittgenstein, 1968, Section 654). We ought to look toward outward criteria, which is why SFBT inquiries as to what the solution will look like: How will they know they have reached the miracle? What will be happening? Wittgenstein's private language argument shaped SFBT's relationship to emotions and the role outward criteria serve in therapy.

SUMMARY

Steve de Shazer and Insoo Kim Berg were influenced by Wittgensteinian thought, and Wittgenstein's ideas played a part in developing and refining their approach to SFBT. Relying on the atheoretical philosopher, de Shazer in particular called upon

Wittgenstein's concepts of language games and a private language. SFBT does not think of language as representational and embraces language as an activity. The founders also relied on Wittgenstein's emphasis on the importance of outward criteria and context. SFBT language games focus on the grammar and context of the therapeutic conversation, and there is no need to search for "something deeper." de Shazer and Berg focused on keeping things simple and helping clients get to their destination in the fastest, most comfortable way possible (Berg & Szabó, 2005). They focused on what worked and did everything possible to avoid getting stuck in a scientific language game. After all, *nothing is hidden*. It was important for these founders to *do* therapy, not *explain* therapy.

REFLECTIVE QUESTIONS

1. What is meant by *doing* therapy and the emphasis on *activity*?
2. How does the private language argument change how we see emotions such as anger, sadness, or joy?
3. How does this model revolve around language games?
4. Why would Freudian psychoanalysis be anathema to SFBT?
5. Why is *nothing hidden* and *everything open to view*?

Keywords

Language Game
Scaling Question Language Game
Miracle Question Language Game
Solution-Focused Language Game
Solution Talk
Private Language Argument
Outward Criteria

Solution Talk Post-Test (inspired by student questions)

1. Do I have to ask the miracle question?
   a. No, Insoo Kim Berg developed the miracle question spontaneously when she was trying to identify the client's preferred future. If you can identify the goal without it, you do not need the miracle question. Just make sure that you are working with the client's preferred future and not your personal goal for the client. If you do use the miracle question, you can make sure your client understands you do not mean it in the context of a religious language game (unless you do). Otherwise, you can restructure the question slightly so you do not use the word "miracle" at all while accomplishing the same purpose. I have heard "an ideal world" instead, for example. Use whatever language such that you and the client *see* what the other means. If you feel you need a disclaimer for the language game like, "This is a funny question…" go ahead and use that. It lets the client know you are going to use words in a slightly different way than they are used to. And the whole point is to be on the same page.

2. When do I use the solution-focused language game?

   a. You maintain your use of a solution-focused language game throughout the session. If you start talking about hierarchy and roles, perhaps you are shifting to a structural family therapy language game. If you start talking about triangulation and differentiation, perhaps you are shifting to a Bowenian language game. And so on. The language you use should be consistent with the context in which you use it. Maintaining a solution-focused language game is the activity of *doing* SFBT.

3. Why doesn't SFBT have a theory about depression and so on?

   a. Wittgenstein argued against a private language and maintained that we do not directly *know* emotions or inner states. I am told it makes slightly more sense in the original German. (He was Austrian). But according to Wittgenstein, to *know* is to doubt, and we do not doubt we are sad, and so on. Being a superfan, de Shazer adopted Wittgenstein's belief. As time evolved and postmodernism developed and seeped into family therapy, a new language emerged to discuss these ideas. "Construct" was a very helpful word. A modern-day social constructionist could say, "Depression is a construct," and a C-DP, narrative, and SFBT therapist would all agree. You cannot see depression. As Wittgenstein/de Shazer said, you only see outward criteria that you associate with depression like tears. Wittgenstein/de Shazer reminds us we need to be careful not to think that language is representational: the language of "depression" does not represent what "it" "is." Wittgenstein maintained that we should not speak about things we are not able to speak about—hence why de Shazer answered the conference attendee's question by not answering the question. de Shazer would likely direct you back to the diary filled with "S's" for clarification.

4. Isn't all the language we use part of a language game?

   a. Yes, exactly. We are trained to use language in context, and we cannot separate language from its context and have it make any sense. Similarly, when we mix up language games, we fall into "non-sense." Remember we have not only the language game but also the form of life in which it is used. You may want to review the table on language games and form of life in the previous chapter.

5. Why do you discourage using a book that tells you what SFBT questions to ask?

   a. How-to books that are not written by primary or secondary sources may get you further away from understanding SFBT. The further we get from primary sources, the more isolated we become from the founders' theories and beliefs. If you maintain your solution-focused language game that sets the parameters of the conversation such that you can be more spontaneous and natural in the questions you ask. I believe therapy is more helpful and joyous the more you can be yourself. If you understand how theory and practice interrelate in SFBT, your questions will follow the "rules" of the language game instead of being something you say robotically by parroting a textbook. Even such a lovely textbook as this one should not be used as a script for what you think you "have to" say. Aim to understand both *what* you are doing and *why* you are doing it, so you do it correctly (according to the model).

6. I still do not understand how language games apply in the real world. Wasn't SFBT supposed to be easy?

a. SFBT is straightforward (but not necessarily easy); everything gets easier with practice. If you have ever shown a recording of your work to someone and have them question your language, but you thought/said, "Yeah, but you weren't there. The client got what I meant"— you're on the right track to understanding language games. Think of the difference between saying, "Yeah, I see what you mean" and "Yeah, I know what you mean." SFBT is encouraging you to say the former. Remember, *just see—don't think.* Do you get each other? Great! You're on the same page. No need to go through the depths of psychoanalysis, etc. Now keep using *solution talk* to get their preferred future and highlight the strengths they have to get themselves there. This is a *brief* therapy model, and you are helping them feel "better," not solving all of their life's problems for them. SFBT therapists are traditionally quick to terminate. Remember in Chapter 7 when the client happened to get a dog and felt better, entirely unrelated to the therapist? Job done. And if they want to come back in the future for something else, they can.

NOTES

1   What is called his "private language argument" involves one of his "mind experiments" which I (SdS) hope to simplify without losing his primary argument. Suppose that my friend Max experienced a private, inner sensation, one that he had never experienced before and for which he had no name. So Max wrote the letter "S" on a piece of paper to remind himself of this unique sensation. When the sensation happened again, he wrote another "S" on the piece of paper. The sensation recurred many times and Max continued marking "S" each time until he filled a small notebook. This notebook is sort of a ledger documenting the existence of Max's private, inner "S" experiences. Now, let's suppose that Max decides to show you his ledger, explaining that he wants to share his "S" experience with you. You carefully look and see page after page filled with strings of "S's." You, of course, want to make some sense of this in order to imagine what "S" must feel like and to share Max's experience with him. But this is a radically private and fully internal sensation, one that only Max has had and which is not marked by any external signs other than "S." How can you make sense of it? All you know is that Max calls it "S." How can you imagine what "S" feels like, since it is internal? How would you know when Max is feeling an "S" sensation in your presence, since this experience has no outward manifestations? How would you know if you had an "S" experience of your own? Is it possible you already did? Might you have a private, inner experience that you think is the same as Max's "S" sensation but really is not? These are the kinds of questions you might reasonably ask about Max's "S" experiences and ledger. If you actually asked these questions of Max, then you would have to deal with the responses, to try and make some sense of them. All of your questions and the difficulty Max has in answering them suggest to Max that he really has no firm basis for declaring that all of these sensations that he baptized as "S's" are the same. Might some be baptized "R" and others "T"? Like you, Max has no external or independent sources for verifying his impressions and memory of the sensations, or for changing his designation of them as all "S's." Given these difficulties, it would be reasonable for you and Max to decide that, despite your best efforts, you cannot share Max's "S" experience and he cannot ever be certain that all of the sensations were really "S's" (pp. 182–183). Without outward criteria, it makes no difference whether or not all the "S's" are the same or whether each one was completely different from all the others. No certainty is possible here. Furthermore, it makes no difference whether or not Max ever really had these experiences. That is, nothing changes for you if

Max did not have these experiences but just says he did. Lacking outward criteria, there is nothing to go on here. Thus, in Wittgenstein's view, the individual does not have special, private knowledge about his or her own inner states and processes. In order for us to talk about, make sense of, and perhaps define, these inner processes, we need outward criteria that can be referenced by and shared with others (de Shazer et al., 2021, pp. 181–183).

2 Section 258. Let's imagine the following case. I want to keep a diary about the recurrence of a certain sensation. To this end I associate it with the sign "S" and write this sign in a calendar for every day on which I have the sensation. ——I first want to observe that a definition of the sign cannot be formulated. ——But all the same, I can give one to myself as a kind of ostensive definition! ——How? Can I point to the sensation? ——Not in the ordinary sense. But I speak, or write the sign down, and at the same time I concentrate my attention on the sensation ——and so, as it were, point to it inwardly. ——But what is this ceremony for? For that is all it seems to be! A definition serves to lay down the meaning of a sign, doesn't it? ——Well, that is done precisely by concentrating my attention; for in this way I commit to memory the connection between the sign and the sensation. ——But "I commit it to memory" can only mean: this process brings it about that I remember the connection *correctly* in the future. But in the present case, I have no criterion of correctness. One would like to say: whatever is going to seem correct to me is correct. And that only means that here we can't talk about "correct" (Wittgenstein, 2009, pp. 98–99).

INSOO KIM BERG AND STEVE DE SHAZER: PRIMARY SOURCES

Berg, I. K. (1994). *Family based services: A solution-focused approach*. W. W. Norton & Company.

Berg, I. K., & de Shazer, S. (1993). Making numbers talk: Language in therapy. In S. Friedman (Ed.), *The new language of change* (pp. 5–24). The Guilford Press.

Berg, I. K., & Szabó, P. (2005). *Brief coaching for lasting solutions*. W. W. Norton.

de Shazer, S. (1982). *Patterns of brief family therapy*. The Guilford Press.

de Shazer, S. (1988). *Clues: Investigating solutions in brief therapy*. W. W. Norton & Company.

de Shazer, S. (1991). *Putting difference to work*. W. W. Norton & Company.

de Shazer, S. (1997). Some thoughts on language use in therapy. *Contemporary Family Therapy*, *19*(1), 133–141.

de Shazer, S. (2005). *Some SFBT language-games* [PDF].

de Shazer, S. (2017). On useful metaphors. *Journal of Systemic Therapies*, *36*(3), 72–80.

de Shazer, S., & Berg, I. K. (1992). Doing therapy: A post-structural re-vision. *Journal of Marital and Family Therapy*, *18*(1), 71–81.

de Shazer, S., Dolan, Y., Korman, H., Trepper, T., McCollum, T., & Berg, I. K. (2021). *More than miracles: The state of the art of solution focused brief therapy* (2nd dig. ed.). Routledge.

Miller, G., & de Shazer, S. (2000). Emotions in solution focused therapy: A re-examination. *Family Process*, *39*(1), 5–23.

Renowned Sources

Korman, H., De Jong, P., & Jordan, S. S. (2020). Steve de Shazer's theory development. *Journal of Solution Focused Practices*, *4*(2), 47–70.

Monk, R. (2019). *How to read Wittgenstein* (dig. ed.). Granta Books.

Wittgenstein, L. (2009). *Philosophical investigations* (G. E. M. Anscombe, P. M. S. Hacker, & J. Schulte Trans., rev. 4th dig. ed.). Wiley Blackwell. (Original work published 1953).

Additional References

Hoyt, M. F. (Ed.). (1996). *Constructive therapies* (Vol. 2). Guilford Press.

Reiter, M. D. (2023). *Family therapy: The basics*. Routledge.

PART V
Conclusion

CHAPTER 10

Interweaving theory and practice

....

REVIEWING WHAT YOU HAVE LEARNED

Part I

The Introduction familiarized readers with modernism and positivism. The chapter discussed psychology's shift from the study of the soul to the study of the mind, moving from exploratory contemplation on what it means to live a "good" life to scientific measurement and explanatory certainty on "mental 'health' and mental 'illness'." It defined empiricism and positivism, two methods of modernist research, carefully explaining that empiricism focuses on measuring what we see, hear, taste, touch, and smell while positivism focuses on following methodologies such as the scientific method to arrive at certainty. It touched upon the "science wars" between modernist research approaches and qualitative research approaches, with the first generally fixated on globalized explanation and the latter generally centered around localized descriptions.

Additionally, this chapter outlined the metaphysical areas of interest, epistemology and ontology, that apply to how we think about the world and ourselves in it. Epistemology studies knowledge (i.e., what knowledge is and how we know what we think we know), and ontology studies being and reality (i.e., what kinds of things exist and what it means to exist). Furthermore, the Introduction chronologically covered constructivism, radical constructivism, and social constructionism, explaining how each of these philosophies contain their own epistemological and ontological positions. A constructivist believes knowledge is constructed based on an individual's subjective experience in the real world. A radical constructivist believes knowledge is constructed in the mind and is not a reflection of reality. A social constructionist believes dynamic social processes, taking place in language, construct knowledge and reality in a shared social context.

This chapter introduced Ludwig Wittgenstein and Michel Foucault, two philosophers who influenced the creation and development of postmodernism, and Ken Gergen, a modern-day philosopher whose social constructionist work falls under the umbrella of postmodernism. It explained the book's reverse chronological structure and introduced the postmodern family therapy models and their founders. Harlene Anderson

DOI: 10.4324/9781003439349-15

and Harry Goolishian co-founded collaborative-dialogic practice (aka collaborative therapy, formerly collaborative language systems). Michael White and David Epston co-founded narrative therapy. Insoo Kim Berg and Steve de Shazer co-founded solution focused brief therapy (formerly solution-focused brief therapy).

Part II

Chapters 1–3 focused on collaborative-dialogic practice (C-DP). The first chapter introduced the model's historical and contextual development from Harlene Anderson's early post-structural work with Harry Goolishian as they moved away from general systems theories and cybernetic "onion-like" metaphors to the growing social constructionist revisions and reconsiderations Anderson delved into after Goolishian's passing. This section contained explanations of Tom Andersen's "both/and" concept, Tom Andersen's reflecting teams, and the "withness practices" made famous by social constructionist John Shotter and family therapists Lynn Hoffman, Tom Andersen, and Harlene Anderson. Highlighting the intersection between hermeneutics and social constructionism, the first chapter profoundly explored the differences between reciprocity, reflexivity, and recursivity, underscoring humans *being* instead of human beings. Chapter 2 outlined Ken Gergen's experience as a philosopher and researcher, summarizing two of his esteemed books and detailing important social constructionist concepts. Chapter 3 explained Gergen's influence on Harlene Anderson's therapeutic practice, including a belief in a social rather than "bounded" being. It connected C-DP components such as conversational partners, "withness," mutual puzzling, genuine curiosity, transformative dialogue, and especially the not-knowing, non-expert stance of a host/guest as having been informed by social constructionist ideas that challenge modernist ways of knowing, speaking, and listening in the therapy room. Overall, this section guided readers on applying the not-knowing stance by understanding the underlying philosophy.

Part III

Chapters 4–6 centered around the narrative therapy practices developed by Michael White and David Epston. Chapter 4 outlined the importance of separating the problem from the person, adopting a decentered yet influential position, and listening for dominant discourses and unique outcomes to build upon the client's subjugated narrative. By bringing in Michel Foucault's philosophy, this section explained how, because of its critique of power structures, narrative therapy's strong post-structuralist ties can give it a stronger political undertone than the other two models discussed in this book. This section addressed narrative therapy's alignment with social constructionism's view of problems as socially constructed narratives based on dominant societal discourses; meanwhile, it clarifies that Foucault's ideas of power, knowledge, and complex social dynamics are more grounded in post-structuralism. Recalling Michael White's focus on the influence of institutions and labels, this section reminded readers that White was a Foucauldian foremost (White, 2012) whose work incorporated social constructionist ideas. Readers learned that although post-structuralism and social constructionism both resolutely fall under the postmodern umbrella, post-structuralism's beliefs in the real effects of power-knowledge could arguably make it a smidgen more modern than social constructionism's stance on multiple realities and that postmodern feminism is similarly critiqued for this reason. This section continued a discussion on Michael White's view of problems as being shaped in language, which shapes reality, explaining that narrative therapy thus overlaps with both post-structuralism and social constructionism. Chapter 6 fleshed out Michel Foucault's influence on White as he sought to deconstruct dominant discourses and stop the objectification of individuals through externalization.

Part IV

Chapters 7–9 covered married couple Insoo Kim Berg and Steve de Shazer's model, solution focused brief therapy (SFBT). Chapter 7 discussed Berg and de Shazer's journey from the first-wave influences of the hypnotherapist Milton Erickson, the philosopher/anthropologist Gregory Bateson, and the foundational systemic family therapists at the Mental Research Institute (MRI) to the second-wave influence of Ludwig Wittgenstein and postmodernism. It addressed the co-founders' formation of the Brief Family Therapy Center (BFTC) in Milwaukee and how, by empirically researching their practices as they started, they inductively formed SFBT. This section's opening chapter described SFBT's basic tenets, key assumptions, and well-known questions. It included a brief comparison and contrast with a model often confused with it (de Shazer et al., 2021), cognitive-behavioral therapy (CBT). Chapter 8 introduced the life and works of Ludwig Wittgenstein. This chapter *showed* rather than *defined* (a Wittgenstein joke) his concepts of language games, family resemblances, forms of life, and a private language. Chapter 9 showed how these Wittgensteinian ideas and his theory of no-theory informed Steve de Shazer's practice of SFBT, which then influenced Insoo Kim Berg's practice of SFBT. Steve de Shazer took a scholar-practitioner approach to Wittgenstein, applying a miracle question language game, scaling question language game, and so on. Tying theory (not Theory) into therapeutic practice, Berg and de Shazer's "technique" of *solution talk* is participating in a solution-focused language game, following specific contextual rules in language to create solutions in a process they describe as "doing" therapy. This section illuminates why there is no need to overly attend to the problem or look for a root cause in SFBT because *nothing is hidden*.

REFLECTING ON YOUR PERSONAL BELIEFS

From the beginning, I aimed to introduce my readers to complex philosophical ideas, making terms like postmodernism, post-structuralism, constructivism, radical constructivism, and social constructionism accessible to readers without a philosophy degree. In Western mental health practices where modernism dominates, universities and supervision sites regularly reinforce that traditional modernist models are superior to countercultural postmodernist models. I hope I have shown that this understanding is based on discourse, not Fact. Modern and postmodern family therapy models each have their own validity based on different principles, values, and measurements of success. Now that you know the intricacies of postmodern family therapy practices, I encourage you to revisit the questions posed in the Introduction:

1. What is the role of a therapist?
   a. *Modernist:* I believe the role of the therapist is to provide expert knowledge, directives, suggestions, or interventions.
   b. *Postmodernist:* I believe the role of the therapist is to collaboratively explore meanings and/or narratives.

2. What is the goal of a therapist?
   a. *Modernist:* I believe the goal of the therapist is to achieve concrete, often measurable outcomes and/or milestones.
   b. *Postmodernist:* I believe the goal of the therapist is to facilitate conversations around meanings and/or narratives.
3. How do you think change happens in therapy?
   a. *Modernist:* I believe therapeutic change happens through a change in patterns, behavior, literal thoughts, and/or perspective.
   b. *Postmodernist:* I believe therapeutic change happens through dialogue and often involves deconstructing limiting narratives and facilitating client empowerment through dialogue. This process creates new constructions of meanings, thoughts, and actions.
4. Should a therapist give advice?
   a. *Modernist:* I believe a therapist should give advice when appropriate.
   b. *Postmodernist:* I believe a therapist should generally replace advice with questions for clients to reflect upon and answer themselves.
5. How does a therapist find out what the problem is?
   a. *Modernist:* A therapist identifies problems through intake paperwork, assessments, observation, and clients' self-reports.
   b. *Postmodernist:* A therapist generally relies solely or primarily on clients' descriptions of what is a problem to them.
6. Should a therapist give homework?
   a. *Modernist:* Homework can sometimes be a helpful tool to enhance therapeutic outcomes.
   b. *Postmodernist:* I worry prescriptive homework may reinforce a more hierarchical therapeutic structure, but clients are welcome to do as they see fit.
7. What should a therapist do if a client fails to do their homework?
   a. *Modernist:* I believe the client is resistant to treatment and/or has another underlying barrier I want to explore.
   b. *Postmodernist:* I believe a therapist should not bring up homework unless the client does, and I would never label a client as "resistant."
8. Should therapists self-disclose information about themselves?
   a. *Modernist:* This should be avoided. A therapist should maintain professional distance and likely abstain from self-disclosure due to the dangers of boundary crossing.
   b. *Postmodernist:* This is a matter of building discernment, not an automatic boundary violation. A therapist's self-disclosure can enhance the depth of the therapeutic relationship, but it still needs to be done with care.
9. What should a therapist's treatment plan look like?
   a. *Modernist:* A treatment plan needs specific, often measurable goals and objective indications of progress.
   b. *Postmodernist:* There is no objective indication of progress, so a treatment plan should have some inherent flexibility built in and be based on what the client believes is progress, not the therapist.
10. At what point is a client non-compliant?
    a. *Modernist:* A client is non-compliant when they resist treatment and do not follow through with the treatment plan.

  b. *Postmodernist:* "Non-compliance" is not a term I use or believe in, and we should not pathologize when a client does not do what we say or want them to do. We should be curious instead.

11. How close should a therapist be to their clients? How close is too close?

  a. *Modernist:* Therapists can be supportive but with professional distance. You are too close if you become personally invested in client outcomes.

  b. *Postmodernist:* Therapists should not be afraid of genuine human connection and ethical vulnerability; these are individuals interacting, after all. However, therapists need to follow ethical codes and abstain from friendships and certainly romantic relationships with clients.

12. What is the function of language in therapy?

  a. *Modernist:* Language is a tool for communication.

  b. *Postmodernist:* Language constructs our realities and can deconstruct unhelpful narratives.

13. Should a therapist use "we" language?

  a. *Modernist:* In general, the use of "we" language is a "red flag" that the therapist is too close and should be used sparingly, if at all.

  b. *Postmodernist:* Therapists may use "we" language to convey collaboration but always with an awareness of power dynamics and potential pitfalls. Discernment needs to be cultivated here as well.

14. When should a therapist terminate sessions?

  a. *Modernist:* In general, sessions are terminated when treatment goals are met.

  b. *Postmodernist:* In general, sessions are terminated when the client decides they no longer want or need sessions.

15. How does a therapist know whether therapy is successful?

  a. *Modernist:* Success is measured by the client's ability to hit certain milestones and whether they achieved the treatment goals.

  b. *Postmodernist:* Success is defined by the client; I should ask them if they found therapy helpful.

Reflect upon which, if any, of your answers have changed. Do you feel better equipped to explain why you are drawn to some models over others? Are you more aware of the intersection between your personal views about knowledge, being, and reality and successful therapy?

INTERWEAVING THE THREADS

Throughout your journey of reading this book, you have learned more about postmodernism and the different epistemologies that underlie major postmodern family therapy models, gaining insights into rebellious thinkers and practitioners. It is important to remember that each one of these models, collaborative dialogic practice (C-DP), narrative therapy, and solution focused brief therapy (SFBT), has a multitude of philosophical influences beyond any one philosopher or theory. While this book introduces the primary postmodern thinkers associated with each model, it is not meant to imply mutual exclusivity. Ken Gergen, Michel Foucault, and Ludwig Wittgenstein cross over with other models. For example, although Steve de Shazer was obsessed with Wittgenstein, SFBT was influenced by Gergen's social constructionism and Foucault's post-structuralism. Additionally, SFBT was influenced by Gregory Bateson's and Milton Erickson's modernist ideas, and so on. Meanwhile, it is hard to find any postmodernist who does not mention Wittgenstein at least once. While acknowledging a confluence of philosophical inspirations, this book primarily focused on exploring one postmodern philosophical pillar per model. The intention behind this structure was to facilitate comprehension, bridging the gap between complex theory and the postmodern "techniques" you will use in practice. I encourage you to further explore primary sources on the models that interest you.

A METAPHOR FOR CONSIDERATION

Inspired by Harlene Anderson's creative "story ball" metaphor, I have created a metaphor to help you conceptualize the differences in these three postmodern family therapy models. In SFBT, the therapist reframes. Thus if we imagine that the client brings in a clay figure, the SFBT therapist remolds the clay and gives it back to the client to see their thoughts and whether they agree. In narrative therapy, the therapist re-authors. Thus we can imagine a client holding the clay while the therapist reaches over, pressing upon the clay, indenting here and there while the client reshapes and remolds the clay at the same time. In C-DP, the therapist practices mutual inquiry. Thus in C-DP, the therapist and client jointly hold the clay. The C-D therapist is not molding, but tracing patterns they see, and asking what the client thinks of them; meanwhile, the client does the same. Rather than focus on walking away with a remolded clay, they inspect and ponder together, shifting "one-way curiosity" to "two-way curiosity" (Anderson, 2012).

CHARTING THE COURSE OF POSTMODERNISM

Postmodern ways of thinking may feel new, but they are not. Author Jack Kerouac's novel *On the Road* contained early postmodern themes such as a rejection of social norms in 1957. By the time Kurt Vonnegut's non-linear novel *Cat's Cradle* came out in 1963, the literary world was officially in postmodern territory.

If we look back to 1957 in family therapy, the "new kids on the block" were the innovative modernists Murray Bowen and the group at the Mental Research Institute (MRI) who rejected traditional therapeutic norms by thinking systemically, with the

TABLE 10.1 Timeline of founders' essential books

Year	Author(s)	Model	APA 7 Book Citation
1985	Steve de Shazer	Solution focused brief therapy	de Shazer, S. (1985). *Keys to solution in brief therapy.* W. W. Norton & Company.
1990	Michael White & David Epston	Narrative therapy	White, M., & Epston, D. (1990). *Narrative means to therapeutic ends.* W. W. Norton.
1997	Harlene Anderson	Collaborative-Dialogic practice	Anderson, H. (1997). *Conversation, language, and possibilities: A postmodern approach to therapy.* Basic Books.

Note. Although the term "essential" is subjective, these are typically recognized as the fundamental books for solution focused brief therapy, narrative therapy, and collaborative-dialogic practice, respectively.

former interested in natural systems theory and the latter in general systems theory. Comparing them to Kerouac, they had a rebellious spirit but preceded the postmodern movement in their field, and their work was still based in modernist paradigms.

Let's look at a timeline of postmodern family therapy founders' publications. We do not see postmodern family therapy gaining traction until 1985, about 20 years after the introduction of postmodernism and about 40 years before the publication of this book.

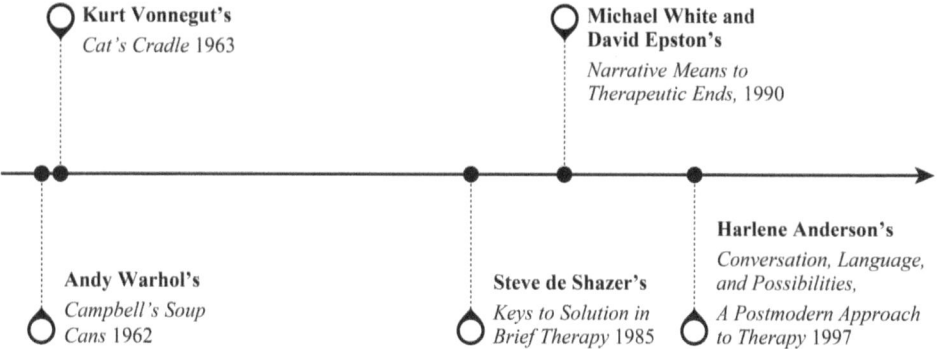

FIGURE 10.1 Postmodern timeline: comparing the emergence of postmodern art, literature, and family therapy

We certainly have come a long way from postmodern family therapy's beginnings. Looking toward the future of our field, I am hopeful that a broadened awareness and more accessibility of postmodernism will pave the way for a wider application of postmodern family therapy models and postmodern ethics in family therapy.

REFLECTIVE QUESTIONS

1. Does modernism or postmodernism resonate more with you? Why?
2. How have your answers to the questions posed in the Introduction changed after reading the book?
3. Are you more aware of the intersectionality between your personal beliefs and postmodern theory?
4. Which model do you find most aligns with your personal beliefs?
5. Consider the timeline of the "new" philosophy of postmodernism. How does this historical context inform how you think about modern family therapy, postmodern family therapy, and future practices?

Key Philosophical Terms You Now Know!

Bounded Being

Cartesian Dualism

Constructivism

Cybernetics

Deconstruction

Deductive

Discourse

Dividing Practices

Docile Bodies
Empiricism
Epistemology
Family Resemblances
Forms of Life
General Systems Theory
Hermeneutics
Inductive
Language Games
Language Systems Theory
Medical Gaze
Metanarratives
Metaphysics
Modernism
Normative Gaze
Ontology
Platonic
Positivism
Post-Positivism
Post-Structuralism
Postmodernism
Power-Knowledge
Private Language
Radical Constructivism
Social Constructionism
Structuralism
Subjectification
Totalizing Practices

REFERENCES

Anderson, H. (1997). *Conversation, language, and possibilities: A postmodern approach to therapy*. Basic Books.

Anderson, H. (2012). Collaborative relationships and dialogic conversations: Ideas for a relationally responsive practice. *Family Process, 51*, 8–24.

de Shazer, S. (1985). *Keys to solution in brief therapy*. W. W. Norton & Company.

de Shazer, S., Dolan, Y., Korman, H., Trepper, T., McCollum, T., & Berg, I. K. (2021). *More than miracles: The state of the art of solution focused brief therapy* (2nd dig. ed.). Routledge.

White, M. (2012). Scaffolding a therapeutic conversation. In T. Malinen, S. J. Cooper, & F. N. Thomas (Eds.), *Masters of narrative and collaborative therapies: The voices of Andersen, Anderson, and White* (pp. 113–150, dig ed.). Routledge.

White, M., & Epston, D. (1990). *Narrative means to therapeutic ends*. W. W. Norton.

Index

Note: *Italicized* and **bold** page numbers refer to figures and tables. Page numbers followed by "n" refer to notes.